IES

How to Live with a Control Freak

BARBARA BAKER

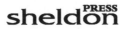

First published in Great Britain in 2010

Sheldon Press
36 Causton Street
London SW1P 4ST

Copyright © Barbara Baker 2010

All rights reserved. No part of this book may be reproduced or
transmitted in any form or by any means, electronic or mechanical,
including photocopying, recording, or by any information storage and
retrieval system, without permission in writing from the publisher.

The author and publisher have made every effort to ensure that the
external website and e-mail addresses included in this book are correct
and up to date at the time of going to press. The author and publisher
are not responsible for the content, quality or continuing accessibility of
the sites.

British Library Cataloguing-in-Publication Data
A catalogue record for this book is available from the British Library

ISBN 978–1–84709–081–2

1 3 5 7 9 10 8 6 4 2

Typeset by Fakenham Photosetting Ltd, Fakenham, Norfolk
Printed in Great Britain by Ashford Colour Press

Produced on paper from sustainable forests

NEWCASTLE LIBRARIES WITHDRAWN	
C460299900	
Bertrams	19/02/2010
158.24	£7.99

Contents

This book is dedicated to the memory of my mum and dad, my grandparents and my great-grandparents. It is also dedicated to my partner Martin Hindley – a very special person

Also to my dear, dear brother, Gary Whelan, and Prue, Izzie and Lucy; Sharon Brown, for her much-valued wisdom, courage, love and enduring friendship, and Neville Mardell; Daphne and John Hindley, my lovely parents-in-law; Susan Carey and Kathy Kennedy for our amazing 40-year friendship, still going strong; Phil, for being a very special person, trying so hard, succeeding against the odds and inspiring me; and Dawn Hastings.

Acknowledgements and about the author

Acknowledgements

With grateful thanks to Fiona Marshall at Sheldon Press, Michelle Clark and Rima Devereaux.

About the author

Barbara Baker is a journalist and BACP-accredited counsellor. She specializes in writing about health, psychology, self-help, food and farming, and lives in the West Country. See <www.journeyscounselling. co.uk> for more information.

Note to the reader

Case studies

The case studies in this book are 'factionalized', but represent typical examples. They come out of my experience as a therapist, a client and a journalist.

Gender

Throughout the book I've used 'he' or 'she' in alternate chapters or sections as far as possible and 'they' where appropriate. All uses are designed to reflect the fact that control freaks may be of either gender.

A word about labels

It might seem that this book is full of labels – and it is! That is despite the fact that I think it's very often unhelpful to label people. First, it makes it too easy for professionals and even friends and family to use the label and see a person as a 'disorder', rather than delve deeper and take the time and trouble to see the full spectrum of the real person underneath. Second, if you're the person who has been labelled, it's not very nice if you feel people have written you off as a control freak (or anything else), because that means they might stop seeing you as an individual with, like anyone else, all the innumerable traits and nuances of personality and experience we all have – positive as well as negative. Also, it can be very difficult to shake off a label once it has been used.

So why, then, is this book full of labels? First, I acknowledge that sometimes a label can be helpful. It can help us to marshal our thoughts and get a handle on different types of behaviour. Second, in a self-help book like this, labels also act as a kind of shorthand, a common language, so we all have some sense of roughly what is meant by it. That means we can more easily access further information and find out about possible sources of help.

That said, I think it's helpful to be mindful that labels often result in generalizations or stereotypes, so even if a label might seem to fit someone perfectly, it's best to see him or her as an individual. It's in that spirit I offer the analysis of types of control freaks (a big label in itself!) given in this book. And in case you were wondering, I'm the first to admit that I can be more than a bit of a control freak myself. I hope that you find this book helpful.

1

Is there a 'control freak' in your life?

Do you live with a controlling man? Someone who always needs to be right, to have the last word and won't listen to your point of view? Someone who always wants to make all the decisions? Someone who insists on knowing how much you spend and what you're buying? Someone who needs to know where you are at all times and what you are doing? Someone who finds it difficult to let you be you or becomes insecure if you dare to have your own opinion? Perhaps it's someone who is extremely jealous, thinks you're having an affair when you're not or even wants to dictate what you wear, who you see or phone? Someone who regularly checks up on you and doesn't believe you, even though you are telling the truth? Someone who becomes angry if you try to stand up for yourself? Maybe it's someone who is just controlling about the way they do things, but their need for order and routine drives you mad! Does any of this sound familiar to you?

Perhaps you're a man with a controlling partner? A woman who has become so strong and determined to have her own way that you have learnt to give in for a quiet life? Perhaps, on the surface, you are happy enough, but inside you wonder how it got to this. Your life doesn't seem your own any more and you feel mad at yourself for putting up with it.

Maybe you work with a control freak. You know you are doing a good job, but this person wants all the limelight or only seems to be happy when he or she is criticizing you or belittling and humiliating you, often in front of others. Maybe you feel you're being bullied and you don't know what to do about it. You feel trapped. Jobs are hard to come by and so you just carry on, coping as best you can, but wishing you could change things.

Perhaps you're struggling to cope with controlling parents, who still seem to treat you like a child or find it difficult to allow you to make your own decisions – and mistakes.

Control freaks come in all shapes and sizes. Often they happen to be the people we love. Sometimes their behaviour is 'hidden' from your friends and wider family because the person concerned seems to be mainly interested in controlling you. To everyone else he or she may seem charming – even the perfect, doting partner – but when you're alone, like Jekyll and Hyde, he or she changes and turns into someone you don't know any more rather than the person you fell in love with or married.

Where this kind of behaviour is more obvious to others than you, you may already have found that people ask you why you don't leave him or her. It's not always that simple, though – especially if you still love the person and still have good times together. It's even worse if you have children. Maybe you think it's just a phase, or you make excuses for the person because you know his behaviour is rooted in a difficult childhood, or he's stressed at work, or it happens 'only' if he's had a few too many drinks. Maybe you think that he will change – if not today, then tomorrow or next week or next year – and that you will be able to change him? You might even have found that, sometimes, you quite like parts of his controlling side – if you enjoy having a strong partner by your side, for example. When you feel weak or vulnerable, then it can seem comforting to know that your partner takes control, makes all the decisions, lays down all the rules. Perhaps you've just given up and got so used to his controlling ways that you can't imagine a life any different. So you just carry on with reluctant acceptance, perhaps even refusing to admit to yourself that this isn't how your life was meant to be ...

This book looks at why people become 'control freaks' and what it's really like to live with a controlling partner – man or woman – as well as how to cope with a controlling boss or colleague at work, or controlling parents. It will help you understand the different types of control freak, how they tick and how to find out if the person is willing to change. You will find plenty of practical ideas and strategies that will help you learn to live with someone who is controlling – not by being compliant, but by being clear about boundaries, so you don't lose yourself in the process. The book will also help you discover if your partner's behaviour is effectively 'psychological abuse' and perhaps help you decide if you've had enough of living with that person. There is a comprehensive self-help section, too, if you think that it is you who is a control freak and feel it's time you did something about it.

2

Living with a controlling partner: what it's *really* like

Is the person you fell in love with, live with or married a 'control freak'?

Perhaps he has always been controlling and you knew what sort of person you were falling for from the very beginning, but decided you'd be able to cope with it or be able to change him. Maybe, at the beginning of your relationship, you even found his control freak tendencies amusing or endearing. Maybe you even thought that it showed how much your partner cared for you.

Perhaps, instead, he wasn't at all controlling when you first met, but it's happened suddenly, maybe after you got married, or had children, or experienced a traumatic event.

Alternatively, maybe it's happened very gradually, almost imperceptibly over a long period of time, in such a way that you've hardly been aware of it until, one day, you suddenly realized that life had become intolerable.

It may be that the control freak in your life only seems controlling in *your* relationship and he isn't particularly controlling with friends or family. Other people might even be convinced your partner is charm personified. He is always helpful, considerate, thoughtful and sensitive when others are around, but somehow changes like a chameleon when you're on your own, leaving you feeling mystified at how he can behave so differently towards you.

Perhaps he is controlling through and through, all the time, with everyone. So much so that perhaps, as a couple, you're quite isolated because friends or family simply can't tolerate your partner for too long at any one time. They might not be explicit about it, but they're always busy if you want to make arrangements or can't get away fast enough if they do visit and you know the real reason is that they can't cope with your controlling partner any longer.

Alternatively, your partner may be just a little bit controlling. It's nothing drastic, it doesn't ruin your life, but, all the same, it's annoying, difficult sometimes and you'd like to do something about it so it doesn't get any worse.

Maybe you're not even sure what a 'control freak' is. What constitutes controlling behaviour and where is your partner on the spectrum? Can you live with it or has it reached intolerable levels? How would you know it has become intolerable? Do you have a sense of what your limit is or are you prepared to put up with anything?

Recognizing a 'control freak'

Let's start by looking at a few core personality traits that drive controlling behaviour. Then let's look at a list of specific controlling behaviours – some of which are very common, others very extreme – that you might recognize.

Typical personality traits

People who are 'control freaks' may have one or more of the following personality tendencies.

- They are self-centred and selfish, often putting their own needs above those of their partners, parents and/or children.
- They think they're deserving of and entitled to whatever it is they crave, whether it's attention, power, respect, money or fame.
- They are highly manipulative and crafty.
- They are deceptively charming, even using humour and wit to get what they want.
- They have double standards – they expect high standards from others and get angry when others make mistakes, but they don't have the same high standards of themselves and don't think they're wrong if they make mistakes.
- They might be good liars.
- They refuse to accept responsibility for their actions and will find ways to justify their behaviour and even blame everyone around them.
- They may present themselves as 'victims', even though they may be bullies or often victimize others.
- They expect support and empathy from you, but seem unable to empathize when you need them.
- They may often be angry.
- They might be attention-seeking people who get what they want by shouting or causing a scene.
- They may be very critical, quick to put you down or try to embarrass you in front of friends or family, ridiculing your efforts or achievements or blaming you when things go wrong.

- They may be quietly controlling and calculating, using subtle, but very effective, controlling tactics.
- Some seem needy and get what they want in a whining, clingy sort of way – they may be masters of being able to make you feel sorry for them.
- They may be 'passive aggressive' types – that is, not openly controlling or violent, but passively destructive and controlling by, for example, giving you the silent treatment, sulking or consistently refusing to show you any emotional or physical love.

101 specific ways in which your partner might be controlling

Control freaks operate in different ways and their behaviour usually falls into one or more of the following categories.

Controlling you by needing to be right and being difficult to live with

He:

- is argumentative and always has to be right;
- always needs to have the last word;
- is bossy and domineering;
- refuses to listen to your point of view;
- constantly interrupts you so you never get your point across;
- sulks when he can't have his own way;
- bullies you until you give in to what he wants;
- won't give up until you agree with him;
- refuses to compromise;
- needs to be in control in order to feel good about himself, but doesn't care how miserable you are;
- can be intimidating;
- may 'use' people to get what he wants;
- if you dare to stand up for yourself, he becomes angry or verbally or physically abusive or sulks, resorts to manipulative or underhand behaviour or getting his own back;
- if you don't stand up for yourself, he may ridicule you for being weak, so you feel you just can't win;
- might cheat at games as he can't stand to lose;
- his need to control puts other people off coming to visit you, so friends and family may refuse invitations for days out, meals, holidays with you or they may leave early as they find the controlling person too difficult to be around.

Controlling you by being clingy and needing constant attention

She is:

- constantly asking you for reassurance that you love her;
- making you feel bad or guilty for wanting to see your friends or family;
- insisting you spend all your free time with her;
- following you from room to room so you are never alone;
- agreeing to go out or do something together and then backing out at the last moment when you've spent time getting ready, booked tickets or made arrangements;
- stopping you from sleeping or doing things you want to do because she needs your attention in some way.

Controlling your freedom

He is:

- questioning you very closely about where you have been – at first these sorts of questions may be dropped into the conversation, but may escalate until he asks detailed questions about what time you left, what time you arrived, what transport you used to get there, who you saw en route and so on, interrogating you because he's trying to catch you out or verify that you're telling the truth;
- checking your phone to see who has called or texted you – one study, which looked at more than 8000 mobile phone users worldwide, found that 1 in 6 people check their partners' phones for 'suspicious' messages, while another survey found that 72 per cent of cohabiting or married women would snoop on their partners' mobile phone text messages;
- insisting you walk with your head down, in case you make eye contact with the opposite sex;
- locking you in the house;
- refusing to give you your car keys or denying you access to the family car;
- forbidding you to see a doctor for an examination, especially intimate examinations, or making such a fuss you end up not going and therefore not looking after your health, or interrogating you after a medical examination about exactly what took place, or accusing the doctor of molesting you or accusing you of 'enjoying' the examination;
- making rules about what you can and can't watch on TV or turning it off if particular people of the opposite sex come on whom he perceives as a threat;

- stopping you seeing family members or friends or even forbidding you from doing so.

Controlling you by cutting off your support system

She is:

- making it difficult for you to keep in touch with friends or family (for example, by denigrating them or running them down) or forbidding you from doing so;
- making visits to friends or family so unpleasant that you feel it's better not to see them;
- threatening friends or family so you feel it's safer for them if you stop seeing them;
- stopping you going or making it difficult for you to go out to work;
- stopping you having or making it difficult for you to have a social life outside the home.

Controlling you by invading your privacy

He is:

- reading your diary;
- reading letters you write;
- intercepting or checking your phone messages, texts, e-mails or post and reading correspondence addressed to you;
- looking in your bag or pockets for 'evidence' that you've been unfaithful or become close to someone else;
- closely scrutinizing receipts, bills and so on, looking for 'evidence' of you doing something that he doesn't want you to do or suspects you of doing;
- searching your car for 'evidence' that you've been unfaithful;
- secretly following you;
- filming you when you don't want him to;
- using listening devices to overhear you.

Controlling you by refusing to trust or respect you

He is:

- regularly or constantly accusing you of having been unfaithful;
- demanding a paternity test to prove he's the father of your child;
- using derogatory language about your gender;
- using or watching porn openly when you have stated you would rather he didn't do so in front of you;
- putting you down in front of your friends or family;

- calling you names;
- not listening to you, continually saying 'whatever' after everything you say, or putting his fingers in his ears when you speak to indicate that he's not listening;
- terminating your phone conversations with him by slamming down the phone or terminating your phone conversations with others.

Controlling your time

She is:

- dictating how long you should take to do certain things;
- dictating how long you can stay out for when shopping or seeing a friend or family member, for example;
- timing you when you go out and making life difficult for you if you are late.

Controlling your money

She is:

- demanding to know how much you have spent and what you have spent your money on and checking receipts;
- refusing to give you money she owes you;
- refusing to give you 'housekeeping' and ensuring that you don't have enough money to get to work or go out;
- taking charge of your bank accounts or checking your bank statements and asking questions about what the entries are for.

Controlling your body and/or how you look

He is:

- insisting that you wear certain clothes or that you can't wear the clothes you want to wear on the basis that they might attract other men;
- insisting that you wear your hair a certain way;
- refusing to allow you to wear make-up or insisting that you wear certain make-up when you are alone together;
- insisting on sex at times when you don't want it;
- insisting that you cooperate in sexual activities that you would rather not engage in, either through force or emotional blackmail (such as making you feel stupid for not wanting to, comparing you to other women or past partners) or else threats of violence;
- examining your body for 'evidence' that you have been with another man – this may include close examination of your pubic area for signs of other people's hair, bodily fluids, smell and so on,

or marks that supposedly indicate you have been with someone else, such examinations perhaps being carried out 'ritualistically' in a set format, such as as soon as you come home from work, or in a humiliating way, where you are abused verbally and/or physically at the same time, or done in a 'throwaway' manner, to make it seem 'everyday' and lighthearted and you may be made to feel stupid for not agreeing to it;

- insisting on showers or washing routines to his timetable or specification.

Controlling you by belittling you

She is:

- putting you down;
- making derogatory remarks about you;
- embarrassing you in front of friends or other people;
- telling you that you are stupid or ugly;
- telling you that no one else would ever want you;
- criticizing you regularly or constantly;
- throwing away food you have made for her;
- throwing your food away;
- sabotaging any attempts you make to get a job, take up study or start a new interest;
- telling you that you are not capable of doing something you would like to try before you have even tried;
- shouting at you;
- calling you names.

Controlling you by refusing to let you make any decisions

He is:

- insisting that only he can make decisions about where you live, where you go on holiday, what car you buy, who you see and so on.

Controlling you by insisting you make all the decisions

She is:

- forcing you to make decisions, but then criticizing you for it, back-tracking on them, forcing you to go back on decisions that you have already made.

Controlling you by threatening serious consequences

He is threatening to:

- leave you;

- inform the police or social services about you;
- tell lies about you;
- leave you without any money;
- take your children away from you;
- burn the house down or damage other things, such as your car;
- get you sacked from your job.

Controlling you by threatening violence or behaving in a way that frightens you

She is:

- threatening to hurt you;
- threatening to lie in wait for you;
- threatening to follow you;
- threatening to hurt a pet;
- threatening to give away a pet without your permission;
- driving too fast;
- exhibiting road rage towards others.

Controlling you by 'punishing' you

He is:

- hiding, stealing, throwing away or spoiling/damaging your belongings or things that are precious to you, such as photographs, keepsakes of your children, family or your childhood;
- hitting or shouting at your children;
- hurting a pet.

Controlling you by being passive, withdrawing from you or refusing to show you physical or emotional warmth or love

She is:

- refusing to kiss you or hug you on a regular basis;
- refusing to have sex with you for unreasonable lengths of time;
- not responding to you by blanking you.

In each of the next five chapters, you'll discover a key type of control freak. See if one of the descriptions fits with your own personal experience. If it does, it may help you to feel less alone, knowing that others have also experienced what you're going through. It might also help you to understand better what makes the person tick, what the underlying cause might be and how you might help yourself.

Each chapter also includes a self-help section to give you ideas, tips and techniques for how to live with that particular type of control freak.

3

Type 1: The jealous control freak

In small doses, jealousy is a normal emotion and very common in both men and women of every age. It ceases to be normal, though, when it crosses the dividing line into what psychologists call 'morbid jealousy'. This is sometimes called 'Othello syndrome' after the character in Shakespeare's play *Othello,* who suffered from irrational jealousy.

The word 'morbid' in this context means 'a threat to health', in this case the person's psychological health. Someone suffering from morbid jealousy is plagued by irrational thoughts and emotions. In turn, this leads to a range of what most people would consider inappropriate and sometimes extreme behaviours, such as the person wanting to know where a partner is every second of the day or covertly following him or her to 'prove' that he or she is being unfaithful.

Jealousy is a common cause of relationship breakdowns. One study by therapists suggested that it was a problem in as many as a third of couples having marital therapy (White and Mullen, 1989). As you might expect, jealousy can lead to domestic violence – and even murder.

A good way to tell whether someone is suffering from 'healthy' jealousy or 'morbid' jealousy is that someone who has healthy jealousy will be willing to change his or her belief in the light of evidence that proves it to be wrong. Someone suffering from morbid jealousy, by contrast, usually won't change his or her conviction, no matter how much evidence there is to the contrary. Of course, not all control freaks are jealous and not everyone who is jealous is controlling, but there is a strong link between the two.

The types of jealousy

There are three different types of morbid jealousy:

- delusional
- obsessional
- overvalued ideas.

From a medical point of view, it is useful to know what type of jealousy a person is presenting with, as this can point to what kind of treatment might help.

Two British forensic psychiatrists, Michael Kingham and Harvey Gordon (2004), have done a great deal of work in this area and identify key features of the above three types of jealousy. It seems to me that all three types can result in controlling behaviour.

Delusional jealousy

A person who exhibits this kind of jealousy regards his views as true – that is, if he thinks his partner is being unfaithful, she actually is, but his fears and theories are extreme. For example, he might think his partner is poisoning him, giving him substances to decrease his sexual prowess or having sex with someone else while he's asleep.

People with delusional jealousy are often very believable. They are so convinced that they are right and present such plausible theories and explanations, that friends and family might even be taken in.

Sometimes this type of jealousy is linked with depression, brain injuries or schizophrenia. It can sometimes lead to domestic violence, suicide or murder (Fennig, Fochtmann and Bromet, 2005). Delusional jealousy affects men more than women.

Obsessional jealousy

The most common type of jealousy, this is where a person may be plagued by intrusive thoughts and start compulsive behaviours in a bid to find 'evidence' of infidelity by, for example, looking through receipts, checking phone bills, looking in her partner's wallet for condoms or continually phoning him at work to check that he is really there and not out with a lover.

Experts tend to believe that this is an obsessional type of jealousy rather than an obsessive–compulsive disorder (OCD – see page 35 for more about OCD). It's possible that a percentage of those with morbid jealousy may have a variant of OCD, though. Professor Gordon Parker (1997), Professor of Psychiatry at the University of New South Wales, in Australia, believes it is important to acknowledge that some people who have morbid jealousy may also suffer from OCD, as many doctors and therapists are pessimistic about treatment for morbid jealousy, whereas treatment for OCD could be effective for those people. Cobb and Marks (1979) suggest that morbid jealousy may be 'indistinguish-able from obsessive–compulsive neurosis' and so could respond to behavioural therapy.

One of the differences between delusional jealousy and obsessional jealousy is that, in delusional jealousy, the person is always convinced she's right in her thoughts and suspicions. In obsessional jealousy, however, the person may well know that her suspicions are unfounded, and will struggle with the barrage of intrusive thoughts she has every day. Much of the time she might be able to resist the suspicious thoughts and keep them to herself – not least because her compulsive checking usually reveals no evidence that her partner is being unfaithful, so she ends up feeling guilty and ashamed of her behaviour. Sometimes, however, her jealousy will spill over and, if her partner realizes he is being checked up on, obviously this will cause arguments, dent the trust that couples need to have in each other and possibly lead to relationship breakdown.

In a way, normal jealousy is a milder form of obsessional jealousy. Someone with obsessional jealousy, however, will put a lot more effort into and spend a lot more time checking up on her partner, and have more problems putting the intrusive thoughts out of her mind. In addition, her behaviour is more likely to cause problems in the relationship itself than is the case with normal levels of jealousy (Marazziti et al., 2003).

Overvalued ideas jealousy

This was put forward by Sims (1995) and others. This is where someone has a firm belief – that her partner is being unfaithful, say – but it is not so much a delusion as a paranoid conviction that she is being exploited and her partner really is cheating on her. In fact, she may even be suffering from what's called paranoid personality disorder (you can read more about this on page 43).

People who have this type of jealousy may also think that other people are against them in some way – friends, family or neighbours, for example – and may generally feel that they cannot trust others.

Causes of morbid jealousy

What causes someone to be morbidly jealous? There are many possible causes and research has come up with many theories, including the following.

- **Feelings of inadequacy** People who feel inadequate or are oversensitive and/or insecure may be more likely to develop morbid jealousy than those with more confidence.
- **Feeling sexually inadequate** People who feel this way may be more

likely to be morbidly jealous than those who have no such concerns, as it can lead to a general feeling of inferiority and insecurity. This can set up exactly the right conditions for jealous, controlling behaviour (Enoch and Trethowan, 1979).

- **Negative childhood experiences** For example, children on the receiving end of their parents' unpredictable rage and abuse may develop a tendency to paranoia as a way of protecting themselves. If they are unable to predict when they might get a beating, or have to endure a stressful or abusive experience, they might end up being constantly on guard in order to always be ready, just in case. The child responds to what is happening to him or her by adopting what is, at the time, an effective strategy. But, as an adult it may no longer be appropriate to be constantly wary of others and could set up a tendency to paranoia – seeing everyone as the 'enemy', even when there's no evidence for that. Similarly, one very small study of just three couples who asked for marital therapy because of the husband's extreme jealousy found that all three men had witnessed their mothers engaging in extramarital sexual activity. It may be that those men grew up with the idea that women can't be faithful because that was their experience as children.

Sometimes extreme jealousy can be a symptom of, or linked to, other disorders.

- **Alcohol abuse** One study (Michael et al., 1995) showed that, in a study of men receiving treatment for alcohol abuse, 34 per cent experienced morbid jealousy, but it may be that alcohol aggravates jealousy rather than causes it.
- **Cocaine use** People who use cocaine may be more prone to delusions that their partner is being unfaithful than those who don't. Regular cocaine and crack users often develop serious problems with anxiety and paranoia, which may feed into jealousy. Cocaine use can also make someone feel depressed, which again may set up a psychological climate where there is an increased tendency for jealousy to occur. It can also blunt sexual desire, and it's possible that this might lead to fears a partner might turn to someone else.
- **Cannabis use** People who use cannabis may be more prone to paranoid feelings that their partners are being unfaithful than those who don't.
- **Epilepsy and other conditions affecting the brain** Very rarely, morbid jealousy can be triggered by epilepsy, brain injury or disease, such as Alzheimer's.

- **Mental health problems** Sometimes, morbid jealousy is the result of underlying problems. Examples include schizophrenia, where someone may experience paranoia or have delusions, and borderline personality disorder (see page 44).

Jealousy and depression

Jealousy is sometimes triggered by depression. Depression is associated with low self-esteem and feelings of failure, which in turn can prompt a conviction that a partner must be looking elsewhere for love or sex. To someone who is depressed and feeling worthless, unattractive and unloveable, and whose mood is so low all the time that she's unable to shake off those feelings, it can seem logical that her partner can't love her any more, no longer finds her attractive and, therefore, is likely to be falling for someone else.

A particular characteristic associated with depression is the tendency to automatic negative thoughts. The running order of an automatic negative train of thought might go something like this.

Jackie and her husband Kieran are at a family lunch when Kieran's mobile rings and he leaves the room to answer it. Jackie has recently been diagnosed with depression and is troubled by automatic negative thoughts. Her thought pattern when Kieran leaves the room tends to go something like this.

> I wonder who's phoning him? ... Why has he gone out of the room to answer? ... That's strange, seems suspicious ... I wonder if he's seeing someone else? ... He's a long time taking that call ... I knew it, he must be talking to another woman ... I knew he was having an affair ... He's finding me less and less attractive and who could blame him? Look at me, who'd want to be with me when I'm so depressed all the time ... Is that why he was so long when he went to see his mother the other day? I thought that was suspicious. My life won't be worth living if he leaves me. Maybe he's already planned to go ... Has he taken his passport ... Maybe I should check ... It's only what I deserve anyway ... Who'd want a wife like me – I'm just a heap of rubbish ... I won't be able to survive if he leaves me ...

Being troubled by automatic negative thoughts such as these is like being dragged down in a spiral of negativity. The person can be so caught up in what she's thinking that she doesn't pause to question the validity of the thoughts, but just assumes that what she's thinking is true. She may even react to her partner as though everything that she has thought or imagined has actually taken place.

There are ways in which people prone to automatic negative thinking can help themselves. Mindfulness-based cognitive therapy (MBCT) could help, for example (see page 59), or cognitive behaviour therapy (CBT, see page 57) and the self-help tips, starting on page 93, may also prove useful.

Jealousy and low self-esteem

Low self-esteem goes hand in hand with both depression and/or jealousy.

Karen says that she never used to be a jealous person, but all that changed when she was made redundant.

Karen

I met my partner Joe when we worked together at a London estate agency. We both earned really good money, we worked hard and we played hard, and were out most nights at restaurants or clubs. There are plenty of glamorous women around in the industry, but jealousy was never an issue – probably because I felt good about myself and had bags of confidence – but then everything changed.

I was made redundant during the property crash and went from being a career woman to sitting around at home waiting for Joe to come home, bored and feeling hopeless. Joe felt he still needed to go for drinks with work colleagues to protect his position at work, which meant I was on my own not only all day but all evening, too. Then he'd roll in very late, sometimes having been to a club.

As my self-esteem plummeted, I found myself worrying that he might meet someone else. I became totally insecure, checking his pockets to find any receipts so I could tally those with where he'd said he'd been. I constantly asked him what time he'd be home, where he'd been, who he'd been talking to, etc., except we weren't even married and I knew that if I carried on the way I was going he wouldn't want to marry me anyway.

He was always accusing me of being too controlling. I think the worst thing was that he felt I didn't trust him, which must have been horrible for him. My lowest point was when I started checking his mobile phone for messages. I suddenly became aware I was stepping over a line I'd never crossed before. I decided that if I put all the energy I was putting into worrying about him and what he was thinking and doing, and redoubled my efforts to find a job, then I'd feel better about myself and get back to the confident person I used to be. So that's what I did. It took me another two months of applying for jobs and failing before I was taken on by another estate agent.

I now feel that perhaps I am a bit insecure underneath, but in the past it never surfaced because I've bolstered it up by having a good career and being lucky enough to be successful. Hopefully the jealousy thing was a blip – that's what I'm telling myself anyway. I don't ever want to feel like that again.

Karen's story shows that, when under pressure, anyone can feel jealous and turn into a control freak for a while. Karen had enough insight to know that her jealousy was a 'blip' and was able to use sheer will-power to pull herself back from the brink.

How to cope with a jealous control freak

- **Tackle the jealousy head on and _talk_ about it** What are her fears? What is she most worried will happen and why? What are her automatic negative assumptions about what you will do? Are they based on her previous experience of relationships in general or maybe just one bad experience? Does she think that her jealous behaviour is enhancing the relationship and bringing you closer together or driving you further away? How does it make you feel to know that you're not trusted? Have you told her? The key here is to have these conversations when you're not angry and she's not in a jealous rage.
- **Increase your feelings of empathy for your partner** Imagine what it might be like for your partner to feel so much fears that she constantly feels jealous and is scared of losing you, fear being abandoned or fears she's not loveable. Feeling empathy for your partner will be a stronger motivation for trying better ways of relating than anger and make it more likely that you can both sit down and _really_ talk about what's happening and how it is affecting your relationship.
- **Don't become secretive** A common response to jealousy is to counter the jealous person's attempts to find out what you're doing or check up on you by becoming more secretive or trying to outwit them – hiding your mobile phone in a less easy to find place, asking friends to 'cover' for you (even though you may not be doing anything wrong) or lying about where you've been in the hope that you sound plausible and your partner stops questioning you. These tactics will only make your partner's jealousy worse. If you are caught out in a lie, your explanation that you were only trying to help her so she wouldn't worry will merely be proof that you are capable of lying. If you can lie about one thing, she'll see it as evidence that you're probably lying about other things, too.

- **Ask her what she wants from the relationship** Does she really want you to be together 24/7, or does she just want you both to have a secure, loving, trusting relationship where, even though you're apart, you are both secure in the knowledge that you both love each other and wouldn't betray each other? Find out what she thinks about how this could be achieved. Are her jealousy-driven behaviours helping you both towards the goal of a loving, trusting relationship or are they more likely to break you up?
- **Draw up a verbal or even written 'contract' between you that sets new ground rules, but be realistic** The Bill of Rights on page 104 might be a good starting point for this process, but be aware that she's not going to change overnight. Her fear and real need for constant reassurance may still be there, so any change will be part of an ongoing negotiation. Keep your expectations low and realistic.

Exercise: Draw up a 'contract' between you

What should you put in the contract? Here are some ideas.

- I won't ever lie or be vague, even if I feel that it's better for you not to know.
- I will be straightforward about what I'm doing, where I'm going and who I'm seeing.
- I'll reassure you of my love/commitment/fidelity on a regular basis, but not to order.

Don't forget to ask for what you want, too

- Make a joint commitment to both sit down and talk at regular intervals – perhaps once a week for an hour – about what's worrying each of you. Take turns to talk for three to five minutes each, with the rule that the other person can't interrupt. Trust will start to build from the moment that you show you believe what she's telling you and feel empathy, even if you find it hard to understand.
- Avoid predictable automatic reassurances that are often dramatic, but meaningless, such as 'I'd never leave you', 'I think about you every minute of the day', 'I can't bear to be apart'. It's easy to get into the habit of saying these things because we feel that it's expected of us, but they will only fuel a jealous person's insecurity if she senses you don't mean them. Indeed, the jealous person might be guilty of doing this more than you, as dramatic declarations can be a way to set up controlling behaviour. So talk about how it might be more meaningful to cut back on constant declarations of love and keep them for when they really are heartfelt and special.

- Make a commitment to take time to have fun, be silly and have romantic nights in together.
- Decide to create some new special routines and rituals. Adopting new routines and rituals at the start of any process of change (as you set out to reduce jealousy in the relationship, for example), can help you both feel straight away that the changes have already started. Be creative about this – always holding hands when you're out, marking Friday nights with a romantic candlelit dinner, bringing her flowers once a month, leaving special notes for each other to find ... These things may seem trivial, but they all add up to create a secure relationship and, in turn, will increase the intimacy between you.
- Consider seeing a counsellor together. Alternatively, your partner may feel that she might benefit from individual counselling.

4

Type 2: The paranoid control freak

When paranoia drives controlling behaviour it almost always centres on a conviction that a partner is being unfaithful. So there is an obvious overlap between the paranoid type of control freak and the jealous control freak I outlined in the last chapter.

Someone who tends to be paranoid may know that his thinking is faulty and be able to reason out his paranoid thinking for himself. Alternatively, he may be totally convinced that he is right in his theories about your infidelity and no one will shake his belief. Any evidence to the contrary will be refuted, ignored or explained away by other theories. He might even go to extreme lengths to investigate what he believes is true and ensure that it's confirmed – turning up at work and confronting you when you're in a meeting with your boss, for example.

Lauren, 24, knows exactly what it's like living with a paranoid control freak.

Lauren

My partner was so convinced that I was sleeping with other men he sometimes phoned me on my mobile 20 or 30 times a day, even when I was at work, to ask what I was doing. It became so embarrassing to take his calls and I was always afraid that I was going to lose my job over it.

His first question was always, 'Where are you?' and my answer was always the same: 'I'm at work, Terry'. If I didn't answer my phone straight away, there was always trouble later. When I'd get home from work it was all, 'Where were you?'

There was no reasoning with him. He would get these things into his head and nothing I said would persuade him that he was mistaken. It got to the point where if I got up in the night to go to the toilet and he woke up, he would follow me. We had a downstairs loo and he would be insistent that I must be going out the back door to meet someone!

He would check my texts all the time, find nothing incriminating because I wasn't getting messages from other men in the first place, but then he started accusing me of having 'secret phones' I hadn't told him about.

I did wonder if his paranoia was connected to his cannabis use as I'd heard it's linked with paranoia.

I began to feel anxious a lot of the time and started having panic attacks. I was desperate to have a baby, but I thought there was no way I wanted to bring a child into that relationship. In the end, I left him.

Although most paranoid control freaks are concerned about their partners' imagined infidelity, paranoia can drive other controlling behaviours, too. For example, someone may be convinced others are deliberately trying to annoy him, or 'have it in' for him. He may withdraw from socializing because he is constantly suspicious of others – and this can affect his partner's life, too.

In extreme cases, someone who is paranoid may use violence or retaliate in other ways against perceived threats or slights, which, again, can lead to controlling behaviours that affect everyone around him.

Jan's partner Patrick was paranoid that their neighbours were trying to annoy him.

Jan

Patrick couldn't see that it was just a difference in lifestyles. Our neighbours were different from us. They were noisy, they had lots of visitors and family turning up at all hours and slamming car doors. It was annoying, but it was obvious to me that they weren't doing it to annoy us – they couldn't care less about us; they were just trying to live their lives.

Patrick started keeping a notebook of the comings and goings of next door and then set up a camcorder to film them. When we argued about it, he couldn't even explain why he was filming them.

If we were in our garden and the neighbours were in their garden and laughing about something, Patrick was convinced that they were laughing at him. He took everything personally.

I told Patrick that if he didn't let me go with him to see his doctor, I would leave him. He was eventually diagnosed with depression and, after going on medication, he did seem to improve.

How common is paranoia?

A 2006 study by the Institute of Psychiatry at King's College London, headed up by Dr Daniel Freeman, found that paranoia is very common, with one in three people in the UK regularly suffering paranoid or suspicious fears. They interviewed just over 1200 people and found higher levels of paranoia than they anticipated – the figures were almost as high as those for depression and anxiety. They found that:

- over 40 per cent of people regularly worry that negative comments are being made about them;

- 27 per cent think people are deliberately trying to irritate them;
- 20 per cent worry about being observed or followed;
- 10 per cent think someone 'has it in' for them;
- 5 per cent worry that there is a conspiracy to harm them.

The researchers highlighted the fact that, in the past, paranoid thinking has been thought to occur only in people with severe mental illness, such as schizophrenia. This study, though, has shown that it's much more common than we thought. It may be that, while more people than we thought have paranoid thoughts, most don't *act* on their thoughts and can manage them most of the time without them interfering too much within their relationships.

It's easy to see, however, how paranoia causes controlling behaviour. The paranoid control freak can drive his partner mad with a whole range of controlling behaviours, which are directly the result of his paranoid thoughts.

Causes of paranoia

In a very small number of cases, paranoia may be a sign of paranoid personality disorder (you can read more about it on page 43). There are some medical conditions that are associated with paranoia, too. These include major illness and diseases, such as brain tumours and schizophrenia. There are also some less severe illnesses that can cause paranoid feelings, such as thyroid disorders, and other metabolic disorders, such as Addison's disease, as well as alcohol withdrawal.

How to live with a paranoid control freak

Someone who is paranoid and thinks that you or others are against him finds it difficult to trust. One thing that you can do to help him, and hopefully improve your life in the process, is to take trust seriously. If you make promises, stick to them. So if you agree to phone or meet the person at a certain time, then keep your word. Be as consistent as you can, within reason, to avoid misunderstandings and engender a feeling of trust between you.

It may be tempting, when under close questioning from someone who is paranoid, to lie or be economical with the truth. You might do this through fear of the consequences of telling the person the truth or to save his feelings, but it won't help! If you are found out or the person senses you really are lying, it will only worsen his mistrust of you.

A consequence of telling the truth may, in the short term, be a tantrum or aggression and you may get hooked into over-explaining yourself and your actions. Trust your own instincts about how much explaining you need to do. Whose need is it?

The word 'reasonable' is a really good watchword to keep in mind and maybe this would be a good subject for a talk with the person. In his heart of hearts, how *reasonable* does he think his demands are? How *reasonable* does he think his fears are? How *reasonable* does he think his actions really are?

Set boundaries. He may not want to see your family for some reason, but is it reasonable for you to stop seeing your family because it helps keep his paranoid thoughts at bay? The paranoid thoughts are his to deal with and should not govern your life, too. Of course, there are ways and ways of refusing. You don't have to shout and protest and storm out. You can refuse quietly, firmly and even lovingly. You can only take responsibility for how you respond. Of course, how the other person reacts may affect you, so it's not necessarily easy to take a step back, but his response isn't your responsibility.

You might be able to model different ways of reacting to situations that could be helpful for your partner to see. If he fixates on something, is sure that something is true, then it could be helpful for you to take a forensic, analytical approach. 'OK, then, let's look at the evidence for the ideas/thoughts you have. What exactly is the evidence?' What is the evidence against? How often have the person's worst fears actually come true? Go through each and every line of enquiry respectfully and individually and show you're taking him seriously.

Where the person's paranoia spills over into worrying about what other people might do in the future or where there is much angst about things that 'might' happen, but haven't happened yet, you might explore how living in the future isn't necessarily helpful as it might *never* happen and, even if it did, is he underestimating his ability to cope with whatever it is? What skills, qualities and abilities does he have that might help him cope much better than he thought? When there have been crises in the past, how has he coped? Did the crises totally overwhelm him or did he manage all right, despite his fears? You might be able to think of examples of situations where your partner coped well.

Help him to look for alternative explanations for things. If someone has ignored him and he is seeing a sinister motive for that, if his belongings seem to have gone missing or he's suspicious of you because of something you did or didn't do, then calmly explore alternative explanations together.

Encourage him to think himself into other people's shoes. If he can see things from a different perspective, that may help him to see alternative, logical or at least possible explanations for what is worrying or concerning him.

If 'vigilance' is part of the problem, ask of what real benefit, if any, based on past experience, has it been to be vigilant? Has it really made any difference? Has it perhaps only increased his anxiety or mistrust?

Ask the person to take a 'helicopter view' of all the times he's been vigilant, on the look out for whatever it is, whether it's your infidelity or something else. Of all those times spent being vigilant, what percentage of them has been successful in catching you out? Chances are the answer will be either 'never' or 'less than 1 per cent'. Ask, 'So what does that tell you? Why would you want to spend your time engaged in behaviour that is pointless and doesn't achieve anything?' Vigilance generally makes anxiety and paranoia worse.

Are they overestimating risks and underestimating their ability to cope in the moment if something does happen?

Is the vigilance taking up time that he could be spending enjoying himself or enjoying time with you?

Has he ever questioned *why* he became paranoid? Was anyone in his family suspicious by nature? Is he a cannabis user and does he know that this may cause or increase paranoia? Maybe being suspicious and wary served him well in the past – if he was bullied as a child for instance – but is it serving him well now or just ruining his life and the lives of those around him?

Is his paranoia sometimes justified? Maybe some of his theories are accurate, but cloud his judgement in other areas. People who are paranoid are likely to be angry if you make the blanket response to his every hunch, thought, idea or viewpoint, 'You're being paranoid'. It will help if you acknowledge the times he's right, too.

5

Type 3: The need-to-be-right control freak

We all know people who need to be right and who are determined to win every argument. They may like things to be done a certain way. Their way is the only way and they won't accept that there is a different way. In relationships, this type of behaviour can be played out around what can seem like very trivial issues.

Alan

Alan has a very traditional view of the roles men and women should play. That's how his parents did things, so that's how he likes to do things. Alan expects his wife Shelley to have his dinner on the table as soon as he gets home from work. He expects Shelley to do what he believes are 'women's jobs'. He sees his role as breadwinner, earning a good wage and doing 'men's jobs' around the house, such as putting up shelves, mending the washing machine, having bonfires in the garden and putting out the bins. That is exactly how his parents divided the chores in their relationship.

If Shelley dares to deviate from that way of doing things, Alan shouts, argues, sulks, moans and sometimes becomes quite aggressive. He has never hit Shelley, but sometimes he shouts in her face until she cries.

The difficulty in Alan and Shelley's relationship centres on Alan's unrealistic expectations of Shelley. First, Shelley works full time and she feels Alan's expectations that she has his dinner on the table and does all the domestic chores are completely unfair. Shelley has responded to Alan's demands by getting up much earlier than Alan – at 6 a.m., an hour earlier than she needs to – just so that she can prepare the evening meal before she goes to work, even before Alan gets up. Shelley admits that sometimes she buys ready-meals to save time but secretly decants them into their own dishes to reheat them, hiding the packaging so Alan won't find out. Alan believes that everything should be cooked from scratch and has a rigid view about this.

Alan needs to be right about everything and, after 20 years of marriage, that's what Shelley has settled for. If she tries to stand her ground, then Alan vehemently fights her and, in the end, she just gives in because she doesn't want to be on the receiving end of Alan's aggression. Shelley feels that she's made a pragmatic decision. She takes the view that her life isn't perfect, but it could be worse if she stuck up for herself. She feels that she can't change Alan – she's tried for years and failed. He's so convinced that his way of doing things is right, he doesn't see any need to change.

Hugh and Tina's relationship is very different from Alan and Shelley's. Hugh is also someone who needs to be right, which has resulted in Tina losing all her friends and being unable to see her family very often.

Hugh is very insecure, but at the same time very dominating. What he says goes. Hugh's reasons for a particular view are often flimsy.

Tina says that it started very gradually.

Tina

I used to have loads of friends and, when Hugh and I first married, he didn't have a problem with me going out once or twice a week with my girlfriends. At first, he started to dictate what time I should get in by, then he decided he didn't want me to go out with certain people. Then he wouldn't have my friends in the house. He also started to make my life a misery about the clothes I wore, saying my skirt was too short or my T-shirt was too low-cut, even though I was just dressed the same as anyone my age. Sometimes, if I was speaking to my best friend on the phone, he'd just take the receiver off me and put the phone down. He started checking my mobile in front of me – he was that brazen. Then he said that I was spending too much time speaking to my sister and she was a 'bad influence', even though I hardly ever saw her.

The final straw was when I got a new job. He didn't want me to work because he didn't want me talking to other men at work. He wouldn't go for counselling as he thought everything was my fault and that I wanted too much freedom, that I must be doing all these things to hurt him and because I didn't want to be in the relationship.

I realized one day that I would end up totally trapped, with no friends and no family and no job or social life if things carried on as they were. Leaving was the hardest thing I've ever done, but I knew it had to be done. Once I'd actually gone, I knew it was the right decision. I don't think he would have changed.

How to cope with a need-to-be-right control freak

One thing that a need-to-be-right control freak may lack is a respect for other people. If it's your partner who needs to be right, talk to her about how her behaviour makes you feel. Does it make you feel disrespected? What did she like about you when you first met? What did she respect about you? Does she respect your right to be treated respectfully? Does she respect your right to be an individual, with your own views and able to make your own decisions about who you like or don't like?

Lack of respect often goes hand in hand with a lack of boundaries. Were the boundaries between you always blurred? If not, what

Exercise: Are you relating to each other as adults?

There is a type of psychological therapy/counselling that is called 'transactional analysis'. It was founded by Eric Berne, whose book *Games People Play* (2004) is a classic and a real eye-opener for anyone interested in how people tick. One idea drawn from this approach is that people relate to each other via one of three 'ego states':

- adult
- parent – there are two types: authoritative and nurturing
- child – there are two types: 'free'/playful and 'adapted'/compliant.

It's healthy to keep moving between these three ego states and adapt according to the situation (for example, you might have more fun on a rollercoaster if you get in touch with your 'free' child), but we can sometimes get stuck in one ego state in an inappropriate way. Where one person needs to be right all the time and tries to impose her will on another, and the other person always allows the controlling person to dominate, then their relationship may be stuck in an unhealthy 'parent to child' relationship for too much of the time, with one partner always the criticizing authoritative parent and the other always the compliant adapted child.

Being aware of these ego states can, in itself, help you to take a step back when you get into conflict with your partner and see what's happening from a different perspective. That may enable you to more successfully shift your relationship by responding to your partner as an adult. A simple example makes the point.

- Your husband, relating to you as an authoritative parent might say, 'You're not wearing that awful top. Change it now.'
- You relating to your husband as an adapted child might say, 'Oh, sorry, I'll change it', even though really you don't want to.

How different might it be if you related as an adult instead? You might say, for example, 'I'm sorry you don't like this top, but I love it. I am definitely going to wear it', staying as adult as you can in terms of tone of voice and being cool, calm and collected.

Of course, responding as an adult won't automatically mean the other person will respond to you likewise, but it might help.

happened to make them blurred? Perhaps at the beginning of your relationship, when you were 'courting', there was more respect and neither of you crossed over a boundary where you tried to impose your opinion on the other, not least because, in the early stages of a relationship, people try harder. Have you both become used to crossing boundaries that you didn't use to cross, such as name-calling, slanging matches? How has this affected the relationship?

Another bit of theory drawn from psychology is Kahler's (1975) work on 'drivers'. Kahler identified five common drivers that motivate us and can cause 'dysfunctional' behaviour. One of these is the 'be perfect' driver. This type of control freak is clogged up psychologically with 'shoulds' and 'oughts', which may be old 'messages' from childhood or how he or she has been brought up. Gently questioning these as they arise might help. What makes you think it should it be like this? What is the rationale? Who says? Of course, it's simply not possible to be perfect all the time. Aiming to be 'good enough' is much more realistic.

Working hard at keeping your boundaries will help, too – just as it's fine for the other person to hold fast to her way of doing things, and have her view. It's OK for you to have a view of your own – you don't have to comply with her wishes: you can both hold competing views and *both* be right.

Exercise: Work at compromise

When you both have opposite views about how you should do things or a decision that needs to be made, try this.

Take a sheet of A4 paper, turn it so that it's horizontal and draw a line across the middle of the page, from left to right.

At one end of the line write on it 'My view' and at the other end write 'Your view'. This represents your polar positions on the topic that's causing a problem.

Now draw two little vertical lines in the middle, crossing the horizontal line, to indicate a middle ground. Make the middle ground quite a wide area to give plenty of room for negotiation!

Take turns to mark a cross in the middle ground area where you'd be prepared to move to from your original positions at either end of the line. It doesn't need to be halfway: as long as you're both somewhere in the middle section, you will already have made an improvement on the original situation.

Seeing it pictorially like this can often really help to underline an entrenched position. What's more, once you've done the exercise once or twice, you can ditch the piece of paper and use it as an instant kind of shorthand between you, as in, 'Yeah, but what's your middle ground?'

6

Type 4: The narcissistic control freak

The word 'narcissistic' comes from an ancient Greek legend. Narcissus was a young man who looked into a clear pool of water and fell in love with his own reflection. He was so besotted with his own image that he would not leave the pool of water and died there.

People who are narcissistic tend to have delusions of grandeur, in that they think they're particularly special or important and they exaggerate their abilities, achievements and talents. Crucially, they have a need for constant admiration and attention, but at the same time find it very difficult to empathize with others.

Often they are very ambitious, have unrealistic aims and what psychologists call an inappropriate 'sense of entitlement' – that is, they think they deserve whatever it is they want, whether it's financial success, power, career success or an idealized love. Narcissists will exploit others to get what they want so have a ruthless streak and, because they lack empathy and feel entitled to get what they want, they may have little conscience about trying to control others.

Types of narcissist

In 1973 an American psychologist, Ben Bursten, put forward the idea that there are four types of narcissist.

- **The craving narcissist** craves attention, is clingy and emotionally needy.
- **The paranoid narcissist** is suspicious and jealous of others.
- **The manipulative narcissist** enjoys manipulating others and finds it satisfying to 'put something over' on the other person, so is often a liar, feels no guilt and has contempt for people. For such a person the need to manipulate is compulsive.
- **The phallic narcissist** is the archetypal 'man's man', says Bursten, whose narcissistic behaviour is about keeping up manly appearances – exhibiting arrogance, preoccupation with appearance, reckless driving or driving at high speed, for instance. Some of these men are contemptuous of women, but may also idealize them as mothers.

Characteristics of narcissism

James F. Masterson, director of the Masterson Institute, adjunct professor of psychiatry at Cornell University Medical Center in the United
States and author of *The Search for the Real Self* (1993), observes that
narcissism and intimacy problems go hand in hand: 'Every relationship involving a narcissistic personality requires adulation and perfect
responsiveness from the partner or an idealization of the partner so
that the narcissist can bask in the other's glow'. When the narcissist
can't get what he wants, 'he resorts to rage which is always externalized
and projected onto the other'. So, if you don't do what the narcissist
wants, if you don't fulfil his needs, if you fall short of being perfect
according to his standards, then *he* gets angry, but *you* get the blame.

Masterson goes on to point out that, while the narcissist often
appears charming to the outside world, if he doesn't get what he wants
he will devalue the person he's living with. At the same time, he cannot
see any of his own weaknesses. His relationships will be superficial
because he is only really interested in others in terms of what they can
do for his ego.

In small doses, narcissism (like other negative personality traits) can
be healthy and work for you in life – provided it doesn't damage other
people or your relationships.

The stalker

Stalkers are perhaps the archetypal narcissistic control freaks. What all
stalkers have in common is a sense that they are entitled to do what
they are doing. What their victims have in common is a sense that
the stalker is trying to control them and has, whether they like it or
not, control over some aspects of their life or, at the very least, their
thoughts. Some victims of stalkers feel so invaded by a stalker's presence or the constant threat of their presence that they begin to change
their routines, are careful about where they go, who they're with, what
they do. They can develop a hyper-awareness of the smallest aspects of
their lives. If you are being stalked, contact the police.

How narcissists control people

Do any of these patterns seem familiar?

- He sulks if he can't have his own way until you back down and he
  gets what he wants.
- He complains until you give in, relentlessly barraging you with
  demands, insisting that you comply.

- He is the master of arguing. He may be highly articulate, able to cover every base during an argument and will exploit any weakness you have if you're trying to stand your ground. Sometimes it's the winning of the argument, rather than the winning of what he wants, that seems to be important. Usually he gets both, plus he might enjoy humiliating you in the process.
- He may be a whiner – whining to get what he wants so you end up feeling guilty or just worn out with his neediness.
- He accuses you of 'betrayal' or 'letting him down' or 'not standing by him' for the flimsiest of reasons. You end up feeling guilty and give in to his demands.
- He uses accusations of your betrayal as a way of threatening that he will leave you, again keeping you closely under his control.
- He won't allow you any privacy. He wants to be with you all the time. He might keep you up talking at night, even when you are tired or ill. His needs come before yours every time.
- He insists on 'keeping up with the Joneses', having friends in high places that maybe you can't sustain financially and don't like anyway.
- He spends a disproportionate amount of your budget on his appearance – new must-have clothes, visits to top hairdressers, designer outfits.
- He insists that you spend your time on activities you're not interested in but he is – sometimes including activities that have a veneer of being high profile, watching Formula One, wheeling and dealing to get access to closed areas or celebrities so he can identify with them and bask in their glory.

Some narcissists don't have to pretend that they are at the top of their game and worthy of admiration and so on because they are in a top position at work or have made it in a particular field, such as sport. Those who don't make it may inwardly struggle with feelings of shame, worthlessness and self-loathing or they may have major anger issues.

Narcissists are typically highly skilled at being manipulative and will use whatever tactics they need to in order to get what they want. Like chameleons, they may speedily change tack to use a variety of strategies to control others. At one extreme they can be whining and clingy; at the other they can be charming and persuasive. They might know they're winding you up or use a system of 'reward and punishment' to control you. They can be good judges of other people's character; in a sense they need to be in order to know exactly which tactics to use with which person. They know how far they can push you and what tactics will work best. Often they're highly intelligent and/or highly successful people, the sort of people who don't mind who they tread on to get to the top.

Amanda believes that her former boyfriend was a manipulative narcissist.

Amanda

Toby impressed me when we first met because he exuded confidence and was reasonably successful in his career as a financial adviser. He earned good money and our life was a whirl of excitement, great holidays, designer everything and lavish lifestyle. After being together for five months, though, I saw a different side of him.

While he did earn good money, it turned out he was also in serious debt. I began to realize that he had no self-control – if he wanted something, he had to have it. He had an inflated ego and if someone said or did the wrong thing in his eyes, he dropped them – there were no second chances.

I felt very stupid when I realized Toby wasn't the man I thought I'd fallen in love with. He was a fantasist who craved other people's attention and he wanted people to envy him and that was often his motivation for doing things. There were times I felt like an accessory. I didn't feel he loved me for me and I began to realize that the way he could turn on the charm was a way of manipulating me and those around him.

I noticed he was often very critical of me. He was obsessed with me saying or doing the 'wrong' thing in front of his friends and I began to realize I often felt anxious about making mistakes or, at the end, even opening my mouth, in case he took it that I was somehow undermining him or humiliating him in front of other people. It was all about his image. Everything else, including our relationship and my feelings, took second place.

He dumped me via a text and I haven't heard from him since. It took me about 30 seconds to get over him. I really wish I'd dumped him before he dumped me.

What makes a narcissist?

Freud was the first person to write extensively about narcissism in the 1920s. He believed that we all experience a period of narcissism as infants when we assume that we are the centre of the universe, but, by the age of about three, we naturally progress and realize we are dependent on our parents and are no longer emotionally attached only to ourselves.

Another view is that narcissistic personality disorder occurs when a child doesn't progress through the normal stages of development because of poor parenting, particularly in response to a main caregiver, usually the mother, who is unable to provide unconditional love and is cold and aloof instead. The child 'searches' for a way to gain its mother's love, maybe finding that the mother values the child's beauty or intelligence. The aspects that the mother doesn't value become part of a hidden self. This split means the child grows up with an inflated view of certain parts of him or herself, at the same time shielding him or herself from inner feelings of worthlessness.

In more recent years, psychologists have linked narcissism with modern cultural and societal trends, too – the rise of the 'wannabe famous' and fascination with celebrity culture, which can give some people totally unrealistic expectations. The booming economy in the 1980s, when people became more money-orientated and adopted a 'live now pay later' attitude, maybe led to a sense of people feeling they could have and do whatever they wanted.

There's also a link here with gang culture, where members may have a grandiose sense of their own entitlement at the expense of others, even others' lives. Some politicians – and, in the case of male politicians, their wives, too – have become tangled up with image and 'style over substance', as well as a grandiose 'sense of entitlement'.

Ironically, the increasingly popular attempts by parents and teachers to build young people's self-esteem, perhaps coupled with the emphasis on celebrity culture, has been partly blamed for an increase in narcissism – the idea that we're all supposed to be happy all the time, and can all have what we want, when we want it. It's all about me, me, me!

How to cope with a narcissistic control freak

Of all the control freak types, the narcissist is the least likely to think that he needs to change, but there are some things you can try.

There's often a mismatch between what the narcissist aspires to and what his life is like in reality and this can fuel increasingly wild or unrealistic projects or ideas. Encouraging the person in what's genuinely achievable could help. If he applies the same enthusiasm and commitment to what's achievable as he does to unrealistic aims, he might achieve more, which in turn would help increase his self-esteem, so making him less inclined to waste time on unrealistic endeavours. When your partner does achieve what he might consider more mundane things, he might be inclined to undervalue them. You can help by praising him for genuine achievements. By the same token, don't fall into the trap of giving praise for planned achievements or wished-for triumphs that you know are unrealistic or involve manipulating others.

You may need to lay down some ground rules of your own about how you organize joint finances. If he's spending too much money, for example, why not keep your money in separate accounts?

Narcissists may lack empathy, which contributes to how he treats you. Find opportunities to talk about *your* hopes, fears, dreams, childhood experiences, so you increase the number of deeper conversations you have. Specifically, ask to be 'heard'. It is quite possible that the narcissistic control freak never really listens to what you want or notices how you feel, because he is too self-obsessed. He may not be capable of listening or being empathic, but at least if you ask for what you need, you're more likely to get it than if you don't bother asking at all.

Exercise: Ask for 'eye contact' time

Gaze into each other's eyes for a set period of time – about two minutes is a good starting point. It sounds crazy, but it's known that this can help strengthen a bond between you. It's what people do automatically when they're flirting or trying to attract a mate.

Narcissists are often masters of arguing and, while that can help inflate their ego, it might be at the expense of your self-esteem and can quickly wear down your morale. Refuse to engage in point-scoring arguments where the only object of the conversation is that he is trying to grind you into submission.

The narcissist tends to look at everyone's situation in terms of what he can get out of it, what he would gain by a certain action or stance or being 'special' in some way. Counter this with your own ideas on what might be lost by that course of action or what might be gained by *not* doing something. Would it really be so bad to not be the centre of attention, not be the best, not be special? These sorts of questions might help uncover the person's deeper-rooted values and what might lie behind his behaviour.

Take a step back so that you are less engaged with his world. What are *you* losing out on by being tangled up in his world? Is it a world that you want to be in at all? What are you neglecting by being caught up in that world? What are you having to sacrifice for him? Don't lose sight of yourself in all this and what your own hopes and aspirations are. Retain your sense of self and your individuality.

7

Type 5: The obsessive–compulsive control freak

Many people can have a mildly obsessive–compulsive personality style or can be a bit obsessive in certain areas of their lives. There's nothing wrong with that. Like the other types of personalities in this book, it's a question of degree and how far it's affecting the person's life or the lives of those around him.

Around 3 per cent of men and women have obsessive–compulsive disorder (OCD). OCD is often confused with – but different from – an even less common disorder: obsessive–compulsive personality disorder (OCPD – see page 46). Although OCD is statistically rare (and OCPD is even less common), many more people may have an obsessive or compulsive 'style', which can lead to controlling behaviour. People who are worried they might have OCD, rather than just a compulsive personality style, would need to see their GP and be referred for an assessment. But the symptoms of OCD versus an obsessive or compulsive style may be very similar. So let's start by looking at OCD.

What is OCD?

OCD affects men and women equally. Many more than the official 3 per cent of people may have OCD, but may not realize it or be too ashamed to talk to their doctor about it, so it may never be diagnosed.

OCD usually involves both obsessions *and* compulsions. Examples of these include the following.

Contamination, germs, illness and hygiene

Fear or avoidance of:

- touching various surfaces, from stair rails to door handles or telephones;
- shaking hands or touching people;
- fear of being 'contaminated' by HIV or other illnesses.

These fears can lead to ritualistic and repetitive, compulsive behaviours, such as hand-washing or body washing, to the point where the skin bleeds. It can also lead to excessive cleaning of objects.

The time taken to perform such rituals may drastically affect the person's quality of life because it leaves no time for socializing and potentially makes it difficult for a person to work or study outside the home.

Checking behaviours

A variety of fears and/or compulsions can result in repetitive or ritual-istic checking of:

- doors – to check that they are 'properly' closed or locked
- windows
- locks
- cookers or other appliances
- cars – that they are locked
- house or smoke alarms
- lights – that they have been turned off.

The person may check several of the above in a certain order, or focus on only one of these but need to check numerous times or a certain number of times. Often he 'knows' that the door is locked, for example, but still feels and acts on the compulsion to check.

Again, this can play havoc with people's lives in a number of ways. The time it takes can make them late for work or college, it can limit social contact and put a strain on relationships.

Jealousy

This can manifest as:

- a belief that a partner is being unfaithful or has feelings for someone else
- insecurity about his own attractiveness or worthiness that leads to a conviction a partner is cheating on him.

This can lead to obsessive checking behaviours, such as reading his partner's text messages or constant telephone calls to see what she is doing (read more about jealousy in Chapter 3).

Behaviours related to luck and disasters

The behaviours stem from believing that bad luck is caused by doing or thinking certain things. For example, that stepping on the cracks in the pavement can make something bad happen, or a casual thought about a partner having an accident could actually cause an accident. The person is then plagued by those intrusive thoughts, which is very distressing.

Another cause is believing that certain numbers, days of the week or year or colours represent either good or bad luck. Lots of people have a 'lucky number' and other such mild beliefs, of course, but those with OCD take them to excess. They find it very difficult to be dissuaded from the belief or avoid thinking about it.

Counting and reading behaviours

These include:

- the need to count things over and over again, whether it's the money in his pocket, which has already been counted, the number of spoons in a cutlery drawer or the books on a shelf
- the need to reread something over and over again, whether it's a letter, a bill or receipt, something in the newspaper.

Tidiness and orderliness

Things don't just have to be tidy, but exceptionally tidy, and very ordered. Books on a shelf, for example, might need to be in alphabetical order or a certain distance from the edge of the shelf or colour-coded in some way.

Another variant is that things might need to all be facing the same way, such as clothes on a rail in a wardrobe, or jumpers on a shelf might need to be all folded and stacked in a certain way.

Similarly, even 'useless' objects might need to be ordered in some way. An example would be old screws that are never likely to be used again being divided neatly into sizes and kept in individual drawers.

Hoarding

A particular type of OCD behaviour involves the hoarding of objects. Sometimes the objects may be of use and value or sentimental value, but other times the items are what other people would describe as rubbish, such as very old but not noteworthy newspapers, bottles or cans.

Some people are unable to throw out anything so their living space becomes impossibly cramped and unhygienic, with every possible surface covered – perhaps even to the extent that there is no room to sit or sleep – with items stacked to the ceiling or blocking windows and doors. Hoarding can also be a feature of OCPD.

Unwanted sexual, violent or religious thoughts

The person may have intrusive thoughts of a sexual or violent nature, such that he fears he might kill or sexually abuse his partner or child or worry he'll feel compelled to jump under the wheels of a truck.

Alternatively, the person may feel a compulsion to repeat prayers over and over again or worry that he will go to hell.

To summarize, in OCD, obsessions take the form of repetitive, intrusive and unwelcome thoughts or images, which in turn may lead to the person being unable to resist carrying out the kinds of repetitive actions or compulsions mentioned above, in order to diminish the obsessive thoughts and anxieties that result if he or she doesn't do them. Some people with OCD have more than one obsession and compulsion at any one time. Sometimes one obsession will fade and another will replace it. Usually a person with OCD knows that their obsessions and compulsive actions are not logical or warranted, but find it very difficult to stop.

Others experience the intrusive thoughts, but don't actually act on them, so don't adopt any of the compulsive behaviours normally associated with OCD. This is known as pure obsessional OCD, sometimes called pure O. Some experts believe that in such cases the compulsions may still be present, but are less obvious. For example, a person might compulsively repeat words or phrases, but do it silently, so it's not noticeable to anyone else.

Obsessive personality styles and controlling behaviour

Someone with an obsessive or compulsive personality style may be controlling in any of the ways mentioned above. It may be that he's only concerned with controlling his own environment, so his actions don't impinge on you at all.

The commonest form of obsessive behaviour in relationships centres on jealousy; a person's jealousy may be fuelled by his obsessive tendency and lead to checking behaviours. Other forms include an obsession with checking things or an obsession with being very orderly, and exerting control by insisting on doing things in a certain way (or insisting that you do) or avoiding doing certain things.

Lydia is finding that her husband Gerry is driving her mad because he is obsessional about keeping the kitchen clean and tidy, to the point where he becomes very angry if anyone else encroaches on his territory. This can lead to him shouting at their eight-year-old daughter if she dares to try and help herself to a drink.

Lydia

The kitchen is like a showhome and I'm happy to leave all the cooking to Gerry because he's a great cook, but I get fed up with the arguments if he thinks that I'm messing up the kitchen or I spill something or put things on the 'wrong' shelf. All the spices are in alphabetical order, he moans if the tins aren't stacked in a certain way and he's fanatical about saving electricity – he insists I turn off the dishwasher *before* the drying time starts!

If I get home from work earlier than Gerry and I happen to be trying to get the dinner on, Gerry will march in and literally take utensils off me and turn the cooker off!

He starts from the premise that I won't have done it correctly, whatever it is, and that his way is the only way. He even tidies nuts, bolts, screws and nails into sizes. It all sounds trivial, but it causes so many arguments. He doesn't think that he needs counselling, so I tend to live by his rules to keep the peace.

Causes of and treatments for OCD

It's not known exactly what causes OCD, but it could be a mixture of several factors. For example, there could be a genetic predisposition to OCD, as it does sometimes run in families, but that could be partly attributed to 'learned' behaviour. Biological factors may also play a part – an imbalance in serotonin (a neurotransmitter or brain chemical) could be a contributory factor, for example.

Depression may prompt the onset of OCD in some people, or there may be other psychological factors at work. Trauma, for example, seems to trigger OCD in some people, but, again, it's unclear whether there might be a genetic, biological or psychological predisposition in such a people as, of course, not everyone who experiences trauma ends up with OCD. So, it's a complex condition.

There are several other disorders on the OCD spectrum, including body dysmorphic disorder (BDD), where a person has an obsessive, irrational preoccupation with his appearance, hypochondria or health anxiety. Some experts believe that phobias are on the obsessive–compulsive spectrum of disorders, too.

How to cope with an obsessive–compulsive control freak

If you think that your partner might have OCD, or he does, bear in mind that, in the UK, there are established treatment guidelines for it that have been produced by the National Institute for Health and Clinical Excellence (NICE). These give information about treatments, including psychological therapies and medication, specialist mental health services and how families and carers may be able to support people with OCD (<www.nice.org.uk>). It's important to understand that someone who has OCD, as opposed to an obsessive personality style, is not doing what he's doing to annoy you or be difficult, but because he experiences overwhelming compulsions that he can't resist, no matter how hard he tries. Knowing this may help you accept his behaviour more easily.

Do read more about OCD. There are many books on the topic, including *Understanding Obsessions and Compulsions* by Frank Tallis (1992). The more you know, the more it will help you to understand the person has a medical condition that means he finds it impossible or extremely difficult to control his actions.

Whether a person has OCD itself or simply an obsessive personality style, it's best not to collude with him in terms of his obsessions and compulsions. Your instinct so far might have been to try and help by playing along with whatever it is he's asked you to do. Maybe you feel sorry for him or it seems to make him feel better and life is calmer if you just give in, but in the long run it will not help. So, talk to him and explain that you will no longer support his obsessions. For example, you won't wash your own hands to make him feel better if you don't feel that you need to, check and recheck doors you already know are locked and so on. It will be very hard to break away from this behaviour if the person has been relying on you to collude with him, so a gentle, sensitive approach to changing tack is best. If the person finds this distressing additional support, perhaps from a counsellor, for example, may help.

Support any progress – for example, give praise if he does manage to make efforts to resist his compulsions. Listen to what he's going through and be caring and non-judgemental as it could be an important part of him making progress.

8

Could the control freak in your life have a personality disorder?

Most people can be a bit controlling at times. If we're under stress or feel a bit vulnerable, if we're juggling too many things in our lives or coping with a major life event, such as a bereavement, divorce, birth in the family, redundancy, money worries or even moving house, then becoming a bit controlling can be a way to make ourselves feel safer when everything around us seems chaotic. We might turn into a control freak for a few weeks or months but, then, as our stress levels reduce, we return to our normal selves.

What about the person who seems to have a 'control freak' personality? She is controlling not just occasionally, when under pressure, but much or most of the time and, crucially, her behaviour is badly affecting her and/or her relationships with friends or family. In these more severe cases, the root may be a personality disorder.

What types of personality disorder are there?

The personality disorders most likely to involve at least some controlling behaviours are:

- paranoid personality disorder
- narcissistic personality disorder
- borderline personality disorder
- dependent personality disorder
- histrionic personality disorder
- obsessive–compulsive personality disorder (OCPD).

Research suggests that about 10 per cent of the general population have a personality disorder (Alwin et al., 2006). The number of people diagnosed with an individual, specific personality disorder is around 1 to 2 per cent. The proportion is much greater if you're only looking at people already in the mental health system – that is, receiving psychiatric care.

To be diagnosed with a personality disorder, a person needs to be seen first by a doctor and then a mental health professional, such as a mental health worker, a psychologist or psychiatrist.

Some people have many of the symptoms *associated* with one or more of the personality disorders and a tendency towards a particular personality type, but do not actually have a personality disorder. In fact, I suspect that most people reading this will recognize something of themselves in one or more of the descriptions here, because we're all multifaceted and certain personality traits are shared by many people to a lesser or greater degree. So, someone might veer towards a narcissistic personality style without actually having narcissistic personality disorder, and the same goes for the other personality disorders. These disorders are really variations on or exaggerations of normal personality traits that everyone has.

If you're living with or have a control freak in your life, it might help to understand a bit more about personality disorders. Even if the person doesn't actually have a personality disorder, which is highly likely, as we know that they're statistically rare, it could be that his or her behaviour is similar to that of someone who does have one. Also, the *causes* may be the same. Everyone, however, is an individual. It's tempting to do an 'armchair diagnosis', but we have to be careful, as labelling someone can just help us to feel superior or righteous or absolve ourselves from any responsibility within a relationship. Where it can be useful, though, is to get a feel for what might lie behind someone's traits and behaviour, as that can help you to understand him or her and cope better yourself. It can also help if we recognize some of the traits within ourselves!

Remember, these are types of *disorder*, not types of people. As stated at the beginning of the book, labels are sometimes unhelpful, but they do provide a common 'language' that professionals understand, and can help with research. This, in turn, can lead to better understanding and improvements in treatment.

To repeat, personality disorders are rare. Some experts do not even accept the idea that there are personality disorders. For the purposes of this book, though, I'm exploring how there may be a link between some personality styles or disorders and aspects of controlling behaviour.

The classifications of personality disorders

There are two main bodies that have provided classifications of personality disorders:

- The International Classification of Mental and Behavioural Disorders was devised by the World Health Organisation and is known as ICD-10.
- The Diagnostic and Statistical Manual of Mental Disorders, known as DSM-IV, was defined by the American Psychiatric Association.

Both classifications are widely used by psychiatrists, psychologists and the medical profession worldwide in order to diagnose personality disorders. The advantage of being given a proper diagnosis is that it can help to ensure that someone receives the right treatment. Of course, some people with personality disorders don't realize that they have a problem, so never seek help.

Personality disorders tend to fall into three groups:

- People with Cluster A personality disorders tend to be 'suspicious' and so include those with paranoid personality disorder.
- People with Cluster B disorders tend to be 'emotional and impulsive' and behave in a dramatic, emotionally charged way – those with narcissistic personality disorder, for example.
- People with Cluster C disorders tend to have 'anxious' personalities – these include those with obsessive–compulsive and dependent personality disorders.

Some things make the symptoms of personality disorders worse – drug or alcohol abuse, anxiety or depression, for example. Also, some people have a mixture of more than one personality disorder.

Paranoid personality disorder (PPD)

Around 1 per cent of people have paranoid personality disorder (PPD). These people have extreme paranoid symptoms and are very suspicious of other people. They may even suspect people who are being friendly as being somehow 'out to get them'.

Those with PPD may suffer from morbid jealousy in their relationships, constantly suspect infidelity and be highly controlling. They can be violent or very aggressive although, inside, they often feel very insecure.

People with PPD can find themselves in a vicious circle – they feel mistrustful of others and are suspicious of you, but, when you refute their suspicions or even provide proof that they're wrong, they misinterpret this as proof that you have something to hide or their suspicions are right.

Narcissistic personality disorder

Around 1 per cent of the population has this disorder. Between 50 and 75 per cent of people with narcissistic personality disorder are men. Some experts believe that narcissism may be a 'learned' behaviour. So, if a narcissist lives with a person he can easily manipulate and control and who, under duress, gives him the undivided attention he wants, then it's hardly surprising that he will carry on taking what he wants if he enjoys exerting power.

A narcissist appears and feels confident and resilient – it's crucial for him to deny weakness of any kind as that would burst his fantasy bubble of everything being OK really.

There's no specific drug treatment for people suffering from this kind of personality disorder. The 'talking therapies' (counselling) may help, though a key factor in the success of such sessions is that of having a good 'therapeutic relationship'. Because of a narcissist's inability to form relationships, that isn't always possible, especially if the person doesn't think that he has a problem in the first place, which is often the case.

Borderline personality disorder (BPD)

This disorder is more common in women than in men, affecting about 2 per cent of the population. It's characterized by unstable relationships, shaky self-image, unstable moods and impulsive behaviours.

Someone with this disorder may tend to idealize some people and undervalue others or may swing between these two extremes – if you're on the receiving end of a 'love–hate' relationship with your partner, then you'll know what that feels like. Because they see things in such black and white terms, they may also have totally unrealistic expectations of you, which can create havoc if you fall short of these demands. They are unpredictable when it comes to moods – very confident one day, yet totally despairing the next, fearing that they will be rejected and abandoned.

Someone with BPD tends to make strenuous efforts to avoid any hint of being abandoned. This may result in pleading with you for constant reassurance. Although this isn't necessarily overtly controlling behaviour, it can be seriously draining on your energy and emotions, as it can seem that no matter how much reassurance you give, it's never quite enough.

In psychological terms, the main unconscious or conscious aim of the behaviour of those with this disorder is a strong desire to avoid being abandoned. They have acquired a range of defence mechanisms to help themselves feel better and cope with life. So, at times a person may be clingy, but she also doesn't want to be engulfed by you, so may appear distant, too. If you are living with someone like this, it can seem that you can't do right for doing wrong. Sometimes if you show affection it may be welcome, while at other times you may feel rejected. This push-pull aspect to the relationship can mean that you feel controlled because you simply don't know what is expected of you.

You can't just be yourself and be consistent about how you express your feelings because sometimes it seems to be what your partner wants, but at other times, you feel you're getting it all wrong and so feel rejected.

People with this disorder may be prone to impulsive behaviours, such as serial infidelity, spending money, substance abuse or reckless driving. Again, this can lead to controlling behaviour, such as holding the purse strings or insisting on driving and scaring you. Anger is another key symptom. Often it is inappropriate – temper tantrums at the slightest excuse, for example – there are violent outbursts or something subtler, such as very sarcastic comments that can be deeply hurtful.

Someone with BPD may have a tendency towards thinking about suicide or self-harming and, compared with the general population, is at increased risk of suicide. In some cases, she may suffer from 'psychotic' symptoms – experiencing delusions, for example, or generally feeling paranoid. It's been found that this disorder may predispose someone to morbid jealousy.

BPD is the most common of all the personality disorders, but it's important to stress that only a tiny percentage of the general population have BPD, and most of those are diagnosed under the age of 30. Sometimes a person with BPD also suffers from depression, anxiety, post-traumatic stress disorder or eating disorders. Some psychologists have suggested the possibility that BPD could result from suffering abuse in relationships.

Dependent personality disorder (DPD)

Those with DPD are people-pleasers and often passive, non-assertive people who may be easily led by others and tend to agree with those around them rather than stand up for themselves.

You might imagine that someone like this couldn't possibly be a control freak, but if you are living with someone who is very dependent on you, very clingy, has very low self-worth, can't make even the most basic decisions and wants you to take all the responsibility, wants constant reassurance, can't do anything without your input or advice and hates being alone, then you may *feel* highly controlled. This may be the case even if most of your friends and family would view that person as the absolute opposite of a control freak.

From your point of view, living with someone who has these tendencies, even if she doesn't have a personality disorder, can be an enormous strain. You may feel that you have limited freedom because of your partner's clinginess and it may sometimes seem like an uphill struggle to reassure her or try to boost her confidence. You might feel bogged down and resentful because you have to make all the decisions and she tends to be so passive. You may feel emotionally blackmailed into staying with her even if you would prefer to break away from the relationship because of her neediness. In all these respects it can feel very much like you're in a controlling relationship that drags you down, even though, ironically, the other person expects you to take control.

Histrionic personality disorder (HPD)

This disorder is almost all about needing attention. When not the centre of attention, a person with this disorder doesn't feel happy or secure. Often people like this are attractive, charming and enthusiastic, but may also be impulsive, manipulative and demanding. Their sense of what's acceptable sexually can be out of kilter, so they may be inappropriately sexual towards others and make attempts to seduce people, perhaps assuming that there's a deeper level of intimacy than there really is. Underneath these behaviours is a desire to please, so they'll tell you what you want to hear, but often what they say seems very general and non-specific, as if they're making it up as they go along. People who have HPD might therefore be seen as quite shallow and emotionally unintelligent. This is quite a hard disorder to diagnose as it crosses over with several of the other personality disorders.

Although it's rare, affecting less than 2 per cent of the population, you may recognize some of the tendencies described above. Maybe the control freak in your life wields control because he's an archetypal 'drama queen'. This control pattern is all about getting his own way so that he can be centre stage and if he doesn't get what he wants, he'll throw a hissy fit until he does. Women tend to be thought of as 'histrionic' but, in fact, there are as many men with this disorder – and these tendencies – as there are women.

Obsessive–compulsive personality disorder (OCPD)

This disorder is completely different from OCD (see page 35). The fundamental difference is that a person with OCD usually realizes that his anxieties, obsessions and compulsions are irrational and wants to get rid of them, whereas someone with OCPD, by contrast, tends to feel that his thoughts and actions are justified and doesn't see any need to change. He may even think that it's other people who have a problem and for this reason usually finds it difficult to make relationships with others.

Symptoms of OCPD can include:

- having a complex set of dysfunctional beliefs that govern most aspects of a person's life;

- being overly preoccupied with lists, rules and minor details;
- having rigid standards that have to be adhered to;
- having rigid thought processes;
- being a perfectionist;
- procrastination and indecision;
- rigid and inflexible attitudes;
- being overly conscientious;
- a sense that 'my way is the right way' or else – anger may result if you don't comply;
- an inability to delegate or share responsibility;
- liking routine and becoming upset or angry if routines are disrupted;
- being a workaholic;
- being very stingy with money;
- needing to be in control;
- having a strong need for order in many aspects of their lives, from how books are stacked on a shelf, to how pens are arranged on a desk, wanting millimetre-perfect positioning; sometimes they might develop a 'ritual' about placing and replacing objects in a pattern or order over and over again until it seems exactly 'right' to them and it would greatly disturb them if someone moved their things; they might need to touch certain objects with both their left and their right hands in a particular order or a particular way;
- black and white thinking – things or people are either all good or all bad;
- regularly finding fault in others;
- being overly puritanical;
- in relationships, having unrealistically high expectations of their partners in terms of looks or other attributes, meaning that they don't commit to relationships or, if they do, the relationships are stormy and unhappy.

Steven Phillipson, of the Centre for Cognitive-Behavioural Psychotherapy, has written a very good article on OCPD, which you can read at <www.ocdonline.com> (an excellent website with lots of information about OCD and OCPD). He highlights how people with this disorder cannot back down in an argument and will rarely 'agree to disagree'. Being with them can often feel like the equivalent of walking on eggshells or, as he puts it, 'land mines', which can cause great tension and anxiety for their partners. Phillipson says that partners can be 'subjected to daily scrutiny and given repeated feedback in a non-loving or supportive manner'.

OCPD is thought to be one of the more common personality disorders. Some research suggests that it affects up to 2 per cent of the population, though one large American study put the figure at nearly 8 per cent.

People with this disorder may have grown up in families where they were highly criticized and mistakes weren't well tolerated, so there was always a need to get things 'right'. The treatment offered for OPCD tends to be counselling rather than any kind of drug therapy, but it may only be effective if the person is able to work with a therapist on reducing his tendency for black and white thinking and accepting that he may not always be right.

9

Causes of and treatments for controlling behaviour

Let's start by looking at the key ingredients that contribute to making someone psychologically and emotionally *healthy,* as this helps us to understand the difference between such a person and someone who has mental health difficulties. Of course, most of us are on a spectrum between these two points, but it's good to have a list of traits or qualities that we can all aspire to!

What traits does a psychologically healthy person have?

A psychologically healthy person is likely to be someone whose emotional responses match up with the challenges life throws at him, so that he doesn't wildly overreact or underreact. He can feel and express a range of feelings in an appropriate way – love and compassion, anger, hurt and so on – and can moderate his emotions, if necessary, without them becoming destructive. He's someone who has self-esteem and a desire and the capacity to move forward with his life, someone who can take steps to reach his goals, is reasonably resilient and is able to cope with setbacks, figuring a way to get back on track without being crushed by the difficulties he faces. He's someone who expects what is appropriate for him and doesn't have a skewed view of what he's entitled to, so he's neither the kind of person who thinks he deserves fame, fortune, success and admiration without lifting a finger, nor the kind who thinks he's not worthy of anything good or positive. He is reasonably self-reliant, not depending totally on others to boost his confidence or self-esteem or sense of worthiness. He is someone who can be intimate in close relationships with others, isn't afraid of some level of commitment and isn't constantly expecting to be abandoned; someone who doesn't need to put down others in order to feel good about himself. Someone who can reasonably find solutions to problems and difficulties. Someone who has a reasonable sense of self and can tolerate his own company rather than only feel safe if he's surrounded by others or being taken care of.

How can all that be achieved? Psychologists believe that 'good enough' parenting and a reasonable set of genes, together with no major traumas (or the resilience to cope with them), is roughly what's needed to achieve all this in one person. In a way, this puts a big onus on parents, as it seems that if we don't grow up in a loving, secure environment where we are allowed to develop and grow in a way that enables us to go through each stage of development in a normal, healthy way, we could end up with personality difficulties. Of course, parenthood is not an exact science and most parents don't have any training for the role, they just do the best they can using a mixture of trial and error, advice and help from others along with their instincts. Psychologists believe that parents don't have to be perfect for their child to have a strong chance of developing into a reasonably psychologically healthy adult.

Some causes of personality difficulties and disorders that lead to controlling behaviour

So why does someone develop controlling behaviour? It's impossible to generalize as everyone's childhood and experience is so unique, but one or more of the following factors may be relevant.

Poor parenting

If the primary caregiver is unable to provide a physically and emotionally safe and secure consistent environment, or doesn't know how or chooses not to or can't respond to a child's needs, that child may grow up without the solid foundation needed to feel loved, secure and able to progress through developmental stages successfully.

Sometimes this happens through no fault of the parents – for example, the primary caregiver may not have been around because of illness, may have left the family home, or died while the child was very young. Equally, it could be that the caregiver was not looked after very well herself and so might have repeated the same mistakes with her own children, not realizing she was repeating the pattern and not knowing how to do things any differently. Alternatively, she might have overcompensated for her own poor parenting and been overly protective, which can set up problems, too.

The absence of an emotionally secure and consistent caring parent or other caregiver means that the child may not properly separate psychologically from the mother as part of normal development. Instead of thriving, the child might feel insecure and anxious. Instead of exploring her environment confidently and learning that it's OK to be separate from mum, she either stays dependent and clingy, afraid of being abandoned, or she becomes distant, learning the hard way that no matter how much she needs her mum, she won't be there for her. She may try again and again to get her needs met and be disappointed every time, eventually retreating into herself because she's learned, possibly from a very young age, that trying to establish a relationship never works. She might even resort to taking comfort from material things – toys or food, for example.

One expert who has written widely about this is James F. Masterson. In his excellent book *The Search for the Real Self* (1993), he writes that where young children are separated from their parents for some reason at this crucial age of development, they experience a mental state he calls 'abandonment depression'. He explains that this is not the same as other types of depression, but one that in adulthood is more about feeling part of the self is missing or lost. He suggests that, in order to cope with life, people experiencing this depression develop a 'false self'. For some this is played out as a personality disorder, such as BPD or narcissistic personality disorder. A child who unconsciously fears that she will be abandoned for being her true self and being independent, may learn to be clingy, passive and submissive due to the misguided idea that it's the only way anyone will love her. Even then she'll want constant 'proof' that she is loved because, deep down, she doesn't believe she's lovable. As an adult, the 'false self' emerges as a sense of self-importance, any faults being denied and a strong sense of entitlement maintained. This is the narcissist's way of avoiding the abandonment depression Masterson talks about. By adopting an 'inflated' false self, the narcissist neatly avoids sinking into the depressive feelings that might more accurately be expected of a child who has effectively been 'abandoned' – at an emotional level – by her parents.

What other factors or childhood experiences might produce someone who becomes controlling?

The child being separated from her mother or father

This is a particularly influential factor if the separation occurs in the first year of the child's life or before she's psychologically mature enough to cope with it. Examples might be if she has to spend unavoidable time in hospital, or if a parent dies.

There has been an enormous amount of research carried out into what's called 'attachment theory'. A secure attachment to a parent is thought to be vital to a child feeling safe and secure. It also provides a kind of 'blueprint' for other loving, trusting relationships later in life.

If that attachment is broken in some way, in adulthood the person may avoid intimacy or find it difficult, because her early experience was that those you love either reject or leave you. It may also result in her finding any close relationships difficult and withdrawing from them, or else seeking out secure relationships and desperately trying to preserve them by whatever means (being hypervigilant about infidelity, for example, or trying to control a partner).

Experience of early childhood trauma

If a child experiences physical, sexual or emotional abuse or neglect, for example, it can make it difficult for her when she grows up to trust other people or make secure relationships and result in very low self-esteem.

A chaotic upbringing

Such a situation where there were few boundaries, no discipline or no supervision of any kind can take its toll. Equally significant is a childhood in which there was too *much* control.

Being constantly criticized by a parent

Never feeling that what they did was good enough, being told that the parent wished they'd never been born, or being put down or often criticized, can damage people's self-esteem.

Having a parent who gives mixed messages

If a parent is one minute showing love and the next minute withdrawing affection, it is very confusing for a child on the receiving end.

Cold parenting

This is where the primary caregiver is unemotional and unresponsive to the child so the child doesn't learn how to show love and feels unloved.

Boarding school

There is considerable evidence that *some* children who are sent to boarding school – particularly if they go at a young age, younger than ten – develop psychological problems or find relationships difficult.

This is thought to be the result of the trauma of being separated from their parents, resulting in deep feelings of being abandoned and plunged into an unfamiliar, potentially frightening situation that feels extremely unsafe, despite the best efforts of parents and teachers to make it a positive experience. A child may try to survive the best she can, hiding feelings of vulnerability, loss and abandonment. She might do this by becoming a 'people pleaser' or adopting a kind of mask or false self.

Some adults who have been to boarding school struggle with intimate relationships in adult life and may even have never really had a sense of who they are. (See Useful addresses, at the back of the book, for a support organization.)

Genetic factors

Our genes may account for up to 50 per cent of our personality traits. For example, research tells us that people who have dependent or compulsive personality disorders tend to have relatives with anxiety disorders (Alwin et al., 2006).

Temperament

Some people are more pernickety than others, leading to a need to be in control – wanting to keep everything just so, for example. Some people just like to be 'in charge' and find it difficult to compromise, which can lead to controlling behaviour.

Brain 'wiring' or biochemistry

This may also play a part. For example, we know that in some cases violent behaviour may be a brain dysfunction problem. It has also been shown that childhood neglect can lead to physiological changes in the brain.

Resilience

It's important to say that not everyone who has had a difficult childhood grows up to have personality difficulties or disorders. Some children are naturally more resilient or able to develop resilience than others. They may be able to tolerate difficult circumstances and relationships better. They may adapt more easily and survive earlier traumas more intact than other children do in similar situations.

There's increasing research being done to find out why some children are more resilient than others and emerge seemingly unscathed from unhappy or difficult childhoods.

Children of alcoholics and controlling behaviour

Children of alcoholics may be particularly prone to needing to be in control of their lives. The Children of Alcoholics Foundation in the United States says that anxiety and depressive disorders are more common in adolescent and adult children of alcoholic parents than in the general population, particularly among women. It's easy to see why this is the case.

When parents drink too much, it can create an unstable, unpredictable environment for a child, with insecurity, tension and anxiety. Imagine coming home from school and not knowing if your mum or dad are going to be in an alcohol-fuelled bad mood or rage, if they'll be sober enough to provide food or care about what you're doing, be able to take you to school, attend a parents' meeting or watch you in the school play. Maybe it would be worse still if they were to turn up – your best hope and worst nightmare all at the same time. The chances are everyone will guess they've been drinking, however well they think that they're covering it up, because they can smell alcohol on their breath, or they will embarrass you or even verbally or physically attack your friends or their parents.

Maybe it's such a secret in the family that you learn not to bring friends home – it's just too risky, too stressful, too embarrassing. You grow up learning to be watchful, adept at spotting every nuance of your parents' moods, spotting a mile off the verbal or physical abuse that could come your way. Even when it's not happening, you're waiting for it to happen because, although everything seems OK now, it will start again very soon, so it's best to be watchful, it's best to be ready.

Imagine worrying so much about your parent or parents who drink that you fear they'll get ill, or die young, or leave a lit cigarette as they fall asleep in the chair. You're meant to go to bed, but you can't sleep for worrying. Maybe you grow up parenting your parents as best you can, checking that they're all right. Alternatively, you might pretend that you don't mind them drinking because telling them how you really feel might worsen their drinking or spoil the relationship you have with them.

People with an alcohol problem are often unpredictable and selfish. The drink comes first. It spoils holidays, Christmas, birthday parties, prizegivings and sports days at school. Indeed, it spoils many other key occasions that should be good experiences for children; what should be happy memories for them as adults are ruined because of it. Maybe they're good at covering it up, maybe they don't bother any more or they lie to your face, again and again. 'I haven't had a drink,' they say with rage in their eyes, daring you to contradict them, when all the time you can smell the drink on their breath, through the very pores of their skin. Maybe, because they happen to be charming, amusing and funny when they're sober, they crack jokes about the drink and you laugh even though you don't think that it's funny at all. In this way you are forced to collude with the very problem that's making your life unhappy or difficult.

In some cases, children of alcoholic parents are victims of sexual abuse or other sexual behaviour that has been fuelled by drink. The parents may dismiss it as inconsequential because it only happens when they drink and is, therefore, very conveniently not fully remembered anyway, so it's easy for them to pretend to themselves that everything's normal. After all, if they remembered, they'd have to face up to what the drink makes them do and that might mean they'd have to stop drinking – a thought that may be harder to bear than remembering they'd abused their own child.

Once again, it shatters the trust that children should rightfully have in their parents. Statistics show that alcoholics are more likely than the rest of the population to be in violent relationships and children of alcoholics are more likely to witness domestic abuse than other children.

It's hardly surprising that children of alcoholic parents may never have had a sense of control in some or most aspects of their lives. Their childhoods have been filled, to a greater or lesser extent, with disappointments, broken promises, fear, anxiety, watchfulness, shame and guilt. Is it any wonder that some of those children grow into adults who are controlling, determined to have the power to control every aspect of their lives in a way that they never could as children? In this way they can ward off the old familiar fears and anxieties that are always lurking in their minds.

Some carry guilt, shame and anger into adulthood, acting out their rage by being violent. Others remain distrustful of people generally. After all, they figure, what's the point in trusting others when they will just let you down? Perhaps that lack of trust will extend to not only their parents but also partners, work colleagues and practically everyone else, too. If they have repeated their parent's pattern and developed alcohol or drug dependency themselves, this will only worsen the problem. Unfortunately, studies suggest that children of alcoholics are themselves up to four times more likely than others to develop addiction problems.

How widespread is this problem? The National Association for Children of Alcoholics in the United States suggests that almost one in five adult Americans (18 per cent) lived with an alcoholic while growing up. Alcohol is a key factor in 68 per cent of manslaughters, 62 per cent of assaults and 54 per cent of murders and attempted murders.

If the person you consider to be a 'control freak' in your life abuses alcohol or her own experience of being the child of an alcoholic is an influencing factor, counselling may be of use. For it to have a positive outcome, however, the person needs to be willing to acknowledge that alcohol may play a part in her controlling behaviour. Unless she seeks counselling for herself – it's unlikely someone with control issues will attend counselling just because other people think that she needs it – it may be difficult for her to change because she may not recognize she has a problem.

Controlling behaviour – could counselling help?

People open to looking at themselves and how they behave, wanting to understand themselves better and maybe make some changes, might benefit from counselling or psychotherapy. These two terms tend to be somewhat interchangeable, though there is an ongoing debate about this. The term psychotherapy may be more associated with a certain type of therapy called 'psychodynamic', which may focus more on childhood issues than counselling does. Sometimes psychotherapy is seen as possibly involving longer, more in-depth work than counselling, but the difference between the terms is much more blurred now than it used to be.

Don't be tempted to think that psychotherapy is somehow 'better' than counselling. Good counselling, whether it's called 'counselling' or 'psychotherapy', often boils down to the individual skills of the counsellor and how well he or she is able to listen to you, feel empathy for you and facilitate your coming to understand yourself better. How effective the process is tends to rely more on these factors than whether you choose counselling or psychotherapy.

There are several other different types of therapies (see the Useful addresses section at the back of the book), so investigate to find the kind of therapy that works for you. Again, whichever one you opt for, it's important to find a therapist you feel comfortable with – having a strong 'therapeutic relationship' increases the chances of a successful outcome.

The very least you should expect from a therapist is that he or she is warm, empathic, respectful and, as far as is possible, non-judgemental. If you get the feeling that the therapist really understands what it's like for you, you will feel 'heard' and that in itself can be enormously healing, even life-changing. It will also enable you to be honest with the therapist and say the 'unsayable', really getting to the heart of your feelings, perhaps acknowledging and exploring your past experiences and emotions in a way that you never have before.

Counsellors and therapists don't give advice or tell you what to do. Ideally you should feel that you are working with and alongside him or her in a collaborative way. They are not experts on your own life, you are. Instead, their expertise lies in helping and supporting you to find solutions to your own problems.

A good counsellor or therapist treads a clearly defined line between being there for you, offering you unconditional positive warmth and empathy, and maintaining a professional boundary between you so that you can feel safe to explore your issues. At the same time, he or she will be very 'real' in the relationship – not just walk into the room and put on a 'counselling hat'! The counsellor or therapist will be human enough to be moved by what you say, but equally will have had enough training to be able to 'hold' any distress in a professional way so as not to crumble. After all, he or she is there to help you!

Another aspect is that good counsellors and therapists should have some idea of what their own issues and imperfections are (they aren't perfect, any more than anyone else is!) and ensure that these don't interfere with the therapeutic process in a damaging way. (That is why counselling training often insists on therapists spending some time in therapy themselves, and counsellors are required to have ongoing 'supervision' with a more experienced counsellor.) Of course, many people are naturally good 'counsellors', with or without training, but if you go to see someone who is properly trained, works to a strict ethical code and has ongoing supervision, it should mean that you are properly protected from poor counselling.

Surprisingly, counselling sessions can be many things – they're not always extremely serious. They can be challenging, interesting, thought-provoking, funny, creative, inspiring, moving, enlightening and life-enhancing, though probably not all on the same day!

What types of counselling are there?

There are dozens of different types. Some of the most commonly available ones are described below.

Cognitive behaviour therapy (CBT)

CBT is one of the most popular types of counselling and the most likely therapy to be offered in the UK within the National Health Service.

CBT is aimed at helping people to identify their unhelpful thought patterns, 'core beliefs' and underlying assumptions, then learn how to change them. People often attribute how they feel or the way they react to an event that's taken place – 'I got angry because I saw my girl-friend talking to another guy', for example – but not *everyone* in that situation would get angry. It's the way an individual *interprets* or *reacts* to an event – in other words, her *thoughts* – that are key. Unhelpful thought patterns prompt emotions and feelings such as anger, anxiety or depression, or may contribute to a variety of controlling behaviours.

CBT can help people to identify any unhelpful thought patterns – such as black and white thinking ('I'm always right') and catastrophizing ('it will be a total disaster if my partner even looks at another man') – that can lead to controlling behaviours. Examples of unhelpful core beliefs include things such as, 'I'm not worthy of love' or 'I can't trust any man' and so on. People often live their lives according to spurious assumptions, too, such as 'everyone should be nice all the time' or 'I always have to say yes to things otherwise people won't like me' or 'it's wrong to ever feel angry'.

CBT therapists work on the basis that the way we think affects the way we feel and behave, so if you can change the way you think, you can change the way you feel, which, in turn, will help you to make changes in your behaviour. Learning to change the way you think means challenging unhelpful or irrational core beliefs and black and white attitudes, and seeing your strengths as well as your weaknesses. Then you can develop more resilience and insight. It might involve homework! You can try out some of the techniques used in CBT your-self in Chapter 14.

Person-centred therapy

This therapy is based on the work of Carl Rogers, an American psychologist and one of the founders of what's called ' humanistic' psychology or counselling.

The core tenets of counsellors working as person-centred therapists are that they view their clients as being able to fulfil their own potential and help them to achieve this by offering real empathy, unconditional positive regard (being accepting and non-judgemental) and being congruent. 'Congruence' means many things, but, at the very least, that the counsellor strives to be genuine and authentic in the relationship.

Person-centred therapists also strive to be non-directive, so the sessions may be far less structured than CBT ones, but the therapy can be just as dynamic, challenging, moving and creative as any other type of therapy.

Many therapists have a number of 'tools in their toolbox', drawing from their training, or ongoing professional development in other types of therapy. As a minimum you should feel that you have had a real opportunity to tell your story, the therapist is very empathic towards you and you really have been 'heard'. All of that in itself can sometimes be enough to bring about some sense of healing or change.

Mindfulness-based cognitive therapy (MBCT)

MBCT is growing in popularity in the UK. Like CBT, it can be very helpful for a variety of difficulties that involve 'autopilot' thinking or automatic negative thoughts or ruminations. It differs from CBT, though, in certain ways. Whereas CBT invites you to change your thoughts to change your feelings, mindfulness is about learning to become more aware of your thoughts and learn that they are just thoughts, not facts. Being more aware of your thoughts in the moment they occur helps you to avoid getting carried away on a train of unhelpful ruminations.

Being more aware 'in the moment' helps you to reconnect with your real feelings, make better choices and tolerate difficult feelings, thoughts and emotions rather than try to avoid them. It can open up new possibilities, too. It can help you to treat yourselves and others in a more kindly way and be more open, experiencing in a new way. Then, crucially, you can tolerate not having an answer, not knowing, not having things all sorted in a black and white fashion, not having things all sewn up.

MBCT has been shown in clinical research to be an effective way of breaking the cycle of recurrent depressive episodes, and it is mentioned in the National Institute for Health and Clinical Excellence (NICE) guidelines treatment to help prevent recurrent depression. A relatively new therapy in the UK, it has been developed by Mark Williams, John Teasdale and Zindel Segal in the UK from the work of Jon Kabat-Zinn in the USA.

The concept of mindfulness stems from Buddhism and is an age-old way of 'being'. The approach is widely used in the treatment of depression, stress and anxiety, and to help people suffering from chronic pain and illness.

You can find out more about MBCT in Chapter 14, where you can also try out some of the exercises.

Dialectical behaviour therapy (DBT)

This therapy may be the treatment of choice for people who have borderline personality disorder.

The therapy centres on validating clients' current behaviour as understandable given their experiences and difficulties, and problem-solving by working through the skills needed for them to respond in different and more helpful ways. It incorporates many elements of cognitive behaviour therapy.

There's a very good article on the subject of DBT on The Priory's website (<http://priory.com/dbt.htm>).

Psychodynamic counselling or psychotherapy

This therapy stems from the work of Freud and other theorists, such as Jung.

Therapists work in such a way that they gain an insight into their clients' unconscious processes and the unconscious patterns of behaviour that affect how they relate to people. Psychodynamic therapists therefore tend to focus more on childhood memories, experiences and dreams compared to, say, a CBT therapist, though empathy and understanding are still prerequisites of this type of therapy, too.

Transactional analysis (TA)

Many therapists use some of the tools of TA in their work, but there are therapists who work exclusively according to the TA model.

TA is an 'integrative' approach to therapy as it uses concepts from humanistic, cognitive and analytical approaches. It was developed by the Canadian psychiatrist Eric Berne in the 1950s and, if you're interested, you could read one of his books, *Games People Play* (Penguin, 2004). TA therapists help clients to look at the way they relate to people and the 'games' people play. By understanding what we do and say and why we make those choices, we can decide to change the 'scripts' we adhere to and learn to make positive changes in our lives.

Drug treatments

If you're wondering whether or not a drug treatment might be appropriate for either yourself or someone in your family, it's best to talk to your doctor.

10

Controlling partners: is it domestic abuse?

For many years, people have associated the term 'domestic abuse' with physical abuse – the battered wife or husband – but it's now accepted that psychological or emotional abuse is also domestic abuse. Indeed, it can be just as serious as physical abuse.

A history of physical abuse is behind a significant number of murders of women, in both the UK and USA. In 1992, according to the Federal Bureau of Investigation (FBI), 29 per cent of all women murdered in the USA were killed by their husbands, boyfriends or ex-partners. In the UK, according to Home Office figures, in 2007–2008, 35 per cent of female murders were committed by the woman's partner or ex-partner. Two women are killed every week in England and Wales by a current or former partner. The British Crime Survey shows that there were 950,000 women victims of domestic violence in 2007–2008.

In some cases, domestic violence is exclusively about psychological/emotional abuse. Sometimes perpetrators of abuse start by using psychological abuse and it culminates in physical abuse. Also, where there is psychological or emotional abuse, the perpetrator usually feels the need to be in control.

It's important to say that, according to UK Home Office figures, one in every six victims of domestic violence is male. Men in such situations are less likely to contact the police than are female victims, and do not have anywhere near the same level of support available to them that women do, so the actual number may be much greater than the official one.

Cultural and social expectations of men are such that many abused men feel great shame if they are being abused by a female partner, making it extremely difficult for them to come forward and report it to the police or seek help for psychological abuse. Even if they do come forward, help specifically for men in this situation is very limited. There are over 450 refuges for women in the UK, but, at the time of writing, less than 10 for men.

The UK charity Refuge, which offers help and advice to women in abusive relationships, launched its 'Early Warning Signs' campaign in 2009, supported by several high-profile celebrities, including comedienne, broadcaster and psychotherapist Ruby Wax, Cherie Booth QC and another comedienne, Jo Brand.

Research commissioned by Refuge highlighted a lack of awareness among women of the techniques used by violent men to control women. The research showed that 95 per cent of respondents recognized physical abuse as domestic violence, but only a quarter understood the more subtle techniques of control, such as jealousy and possessiveness, as indicators of domestic violence. Of the women who took part in the study, 50 per cent said that they had experienced at least one of the warning signs, but of these only one fifth said that they would talk to someone about the abuse.

Sandra Horley, OBE, chief executive of Refuge, said:

> Two women are killed every week by a current or former partner. This is a huge statistic and one that we need to start addressing. … It is essential that women receive the right education and information so they can understand the techniques of control frequently used by abusive men. It's all too easy for women to excuse their partner's possessive and jealous behaviour – but in so doing, they run the risk of the abuse increasing in frequency and severity over time. By understanding the signs early, a woman is forewarned and forearmed.

Signs that your partner is controlling you

- He is jealous and possessive.
- He cuts you off from family and friends and tries to isolate you.
- He is charming one minute and abusive the next, with sudden changes of mood.
- He controls your life – your money, who you should see, what you should wear, for example.
- He monitors your movements.
- He blames you for the abuse.
- He humiliates or insults you in front of others.
- He verbally abuses you.
- He constantly criticizes you.
- He uses anger and intimidation to frighten you and make you comply with his demands.
- He tells you that you are useless and couldn't cope without him.
- He threatens to hurt you or people close to you if you leave him.

- You end up changing your behaviour to avoid making him angry and triggering an attack.
- He forces you to have sex when you don't want to.

There are many other ways in which someone can be abusive. Here are some examples:

- damaging your possessions or threatening to
- smashing up furniture or household items
- destroying personal mementos that he knows are important to you
- threatening to injure or kill your pets
- threatening to get custody of the children if you leave
- locking you out of the house during an argument
- terrorizing you by driving too fast because he knows that it frightens you.

The aim of all these behaviours is to take control of your life and maintain power over you.

Studies have shown that women or men who abuse their partners psychologically use a variety of controlling tactics, which can result in mental distress. They may, for example:

- belittle you either when you are alone together or in front of other people;
- check up on you to try and catch you out;
- isolate you – this may be done systematically over a period of time so that you are slowly cut off from friends and family and become psychologically and possibly financially dependent on your partner;
- tell you what to do, who you can and cannot see, what you can wear, who you can and cannot phone;
- call you names;
- demand that you do what they say;
- treat you like a servant;
- force you to have sex when you don't feel like it or rape you;
- refuse to let you take a job or make it very difficult for you to do so;
- refuse to let you study or have interests outside the home or make this very difficult;
- insist on sexual activities that you don't want to do or participate in.

Sometimes mental and emotional abuse can be a prelude to physical violence, sometimes it happens along with physical violence, while other times it can start when the perpetrator for some reason stops using physical violence, but may see psychological abuse as 'more acceptable'. A study by Dutton and Painter (1993) indicates that most women who are physically abused also report psychological abuse and another (Follingstad et al., 1990) suggests that 99 per cent of battered women have experienced some form of emotional abuse. Not all women who are psychologically abused suffer physical abuse, but psychological abuse may be a reliable predictor that physical abuse could follow at some point.

As psychological abuse tends to be more 'hidden' than physical abuse (though, of course, physical abuse can be, too), there has been far less research in this area than is the case for physical abuse. One of the key researchers who has done work in this field, though, is Linda Marshall from the University of Texas. She highlights the fact that psychological abuse can, broadly speaking, be either 'overt' (obvious) or 'subtle'. She says that examples of overt psychological abuse include instances of a partner trying to:

- dominate – trying to get you to say you were wrong even if you think you were right, for example;
- exhibit indifference – such as ignoring you;
- monitor you – check up on you;
- discredit you – try to make you look bad in front of others, for instance.

Subtle psychological abuse, says Marshall, includes times when he will do the following:

- undermine you – make you feel ashamed of yourself, for example;
- discount you – for example, act like there's something wrong with you mentally;
- isolate you – making it difficult for you to have your own friends.

All the above forms of psychological abuse, whether overt or subtle, can involve behaviour that is controlling in one way or another.

In her research, Marshall makes the acute observation that some abusers, as well as trying to keep their partners away from others, may also try to keep their victims isolated from themselves, by restricting the amount of time they are allowed to be on their own with their own thoughts and just enjoy their own private moments. So they would not even have the luxury of 'thinking time' to reflect on what was happening and perhaps conclude that the relationship wasn't healthy and, indeed, was highly damaging.

She also points out that even the most violent men sometimes inflict subtle types of psychological abuse and are 'gentle and loving' while they are doing it. This is an important finding as it helps us to realize that psychological abuse doesn't have to be delivered in an aggressive, domineering, overtly controlling way. It can be done very subtly, but still be very controlling.

Angie lived with her boyfriend for four years. In that time she went from being part of a loving family, with a mum she got on well with and a younger brother who doted on her, to not being able to see them because her boyfriend Rick didn't want her to.

Angie says that he never actually told her she couldn't see them.

Angie

He didn't forbid me – in fact, sometimes he even suggested I went to see them – which, as I look back, I find confusing, because, at the time, it was absolutely clear that there was no way I could see them because I knew it would result in him being horrible to me. I was made to feel there was something wrong with me for wanting to see them. It was only when my brother was attacked in the street that I knew it had to stop. Rick made me feel guilty for wanting to visit my brother in hospital. For once, I was absolutely certain in my own mind that this was wrong. Standing up to him and visiting my brother in hospital was the turning point. It gave me space away from him, a place where he wouldn't come, and I had the time and space to realize I wanted to end the relationship and that's what I did.

Some effects of psychological abuse

Crucially, several studies suggest that the effects of psychological abuse are just as damaging – or even more damaging – than the effects of physical abuse.

What types of psychological abuse do victims find the most damaging? One study (Follingstad et al., 1990) found that being ridiculed was the worst – probably because it undermines a person's sense of self and results in low self-esteem. Another found that being dominated and isolated from friends and family was the worst (Dutton and Painter, 1993).

Of course, even where abuse is solely physical, there is much evidence to show that this can have damaging psychological effects, too, including anxiety, depression and attempted or actual suicide (Arias and Pape, 1999). Unfortunately, few studies have separated out the two types of abuse and studied their relative impacts on mental health. One startling finding, though, is that women on the receiving end of abuse, whether physical or psychological, are likely to show symptoms of post-traumatic stress disorder (PTSD). The estimates of the numbers of abused women (the research focused on women so there are no figures for abused men) showing symptoms of PTSD vary between 33 and 84 per cent (Arias and Pape, 1999). Crucially, the researchers suggest that the symptoms of PTSD may be 'stressful enough to interfere with women's attempts to escape abusive relationships'.

PTSD is normally associated with people who have had a single or series of traumatic events happen to them. This could be a car accident, rape, life-threatening accident, witnessing something horrific, such as a violent death or being in military combat, being involved in a traumatic event, such as a natural disaster, being taken hostage or being diagnosed with a life-threatening illness.

Typical symptoms of PTSD include:

- avoidance of anything that reminds them of the trauma that they have endured – not talking or thinking about it, expressing feelings about it and so on;
- intrusion of memories of the trauma, including flashbacks and nightmares about the event;
- feeling numb and/or 'detached' from what's happened – a kind of 'disassociation', which is a way of trying to avoid any pain associated with the event;
- hypervigilance – a need to be constantly on alert, as though looking out for danger, feeling jumpy or constantly tense, as though waiting for something to happen;
- feeling irritable, anxious or panicky and/or experiencing mood swings;
- difficulty sleeping and/or nightmares;
- difficulty concentrating;
- depression;
- drinking too much alcohol;
- experiencing a range of physical symptoms that don't seem to have any other cause, such as aches, pains, headaches, stomach problems;
- feelings of shame and guilt, as well as numbness to the point where they don't 'feel' anything at all, perhaps feeling cut off from everything and everyone around them, unable to enjoy anything very much at all.

Arias and Pape found that where women showed symptoms of PTSD, this reduced the chances of them ending the relationship – no matter how badly they were being treated. This suggests to me that perhaps there is a 'tipping point' – that once psychological abuse is ingrained, once it is severe or prolonged enough to cause the symptoms of

PTSD, then they may be less likely to have the necessary strength, self-esteem or resilience to make the decision to leave the relationship, because the trauma of being psychologically abused has wiped out their reserves of these qualities.

In recent years there has been an increase in the amount of research carried out into psychological abuse. These are some of the findings.

- In a study of 578 women who had been in long-term 'bad or stressful' relationships with men, 97 per cent had experienced psychological abuse and 87 per cent had been physically assaulted by their partners (Marshall, 1996).
- A study of 145 women in Italy who had contacted a battered women's shelter (Baldry, 2003) showed that they reported a relatively high frequency of abuse, especially psychological abuse. Most of the women suffered 'often' or 'very often' from being 'degraded, insulted and controlled'. The study found that the women who were psychologically abused suffered symptoms such as anxiety and depression and low self-esteem.
- Women who endure psychological abuse tend to suffer more frequently than average from serious or chronic illnesses (Marshall, 1996).
- Victims of psychological abuse tend to have low self-esteem and often find the experience of psychological abuse even more difficult to endure than physical abuse. They also experience anxiety, depression, feelings of shame and fear of their partner (Aguilar and Nightingale, 1994).

Stockholm syndrome

The term 'Stockholm syndrome' was devised in the 1970s, when it was discovered that hostages taken during a bank robbery in Stockholm had become emotionally attached to the people who had taken them hostage, and even defended their actions when the ordeal was over. Some researchers though (Graham et al., 1994), have used the term to describe the way some victims of psychological abuse within relationships, in a sense, suffer from Stockholm syndrome, as they tend to identify with the perpetrators when they are being 'kind' and deny to both themselves and others that they are being abused or feel afraid, even though they may literally be at the mercy of their partners.

It's almost as though they have become conditioned to the abuse, to the point where they see it as normal or even justify it. This can help abusers to keep their victims isolated from family and friends, as they may become so conditioned to the abuse that they unwittingly become the mouthpiece of their abusers.

This may partly account for the fact that victims of abuse often don't leave the abusive relationships, much to the frustration of family and friends. Of course, sometimes it's because they are afraid to, don't know how to, or haven't got the financial wherewithal to do so or somewhere to go, but sometimes it's because they don't actually realize just how abusive and destructive the relationship is. Even if they do, they can't admit it to themselves. One thing is for sure, leaving an abusive relationship is rarely simple, for a variety of reasons. It can be easy for those who look on to say 'just leave him' or 'just leave her', but relationships, feelings, choices, changes and big decisions are always difficult and abusive relationships can be even more complex.

Extreme forms of this type of relationship could fit into what has been called the theory of 'traumatic bonding' (a term coined by two psychologists, Dutton and Painter, in 1993). In their paper about Stockholm syndrome, Graham et al. (1994) suggested that two factors are key to the formation of this type of emotional attachment:

- a power imbalance in the relationship
- on, off, good and bad treatment by the perpetrator.

It's this type of nice and nasty treatment that keeps some couples codependent on each other. Meanwhile, the victim's self-esteem typically plummets and research suggests that the more a person is on the receiving end of psychological abuse, the less self-esteem she will have, making it more difficult to leave.

It's easy to see from this how women who are with someone who is psychologically controlling – nasty to her when he doesn't get what he wants and nice when he does – may conclude that trying to please him actually works because, look, he's being kind to her again. Graham suggests that some women may unconsciously realize that loving their partner more is a way to reduce the amount of abuse that is directed towards them. Sadly, this just keeps them locked into their abusive relationships.

If you are in an abusive relationship, of whatever kind, consider getting some support. See the Useful addresses section at the back of the book.

11

How to live with a control freak: survival tactics

Ask yourself the sixty-four thousand dollar question: can someone who is very controlling change, regardless of what is causing the behaviour? The answer is undoubtedly yes – but only if that person is open to looking at herself and motivated to do something about it. The bottom line is this: *you can't make someone change unless she wants to do it for herself.*

If she doesn't think that she needs to change or doesn't want to try, you have three choices:

- You can put up with things exactly as they are.
- You can change the way you view and cope with her behaviour.
- You can end your relationship with her.

At the very least, you might want to talk to her and tell her how her behaviour is affecting you. You've probably tried this already, but in case you haven't or you want to try something new, the following ideas and strategies might help.

Find out if she is willing to change

- Start by telling her how you feel. It's best to do this when you're not in the midst of an argument.
- Defuse tension by beginning sentences with 'I feel ...' statements, so that you're owning how *you* feel rather than making accusations about her behaviour.
- Ask for what you want and explain the difference it would make to you and the possible beneficial effects it might have on the relationship.
- Ask if she would like to make changes for herself (rather than just to please you). What difference would it make to her life from her own perspective? Is she really happy to continue as she is?
- Ask how you could support her. Are there changes you would be willing to make (other than colluding with her controlling behaviour) that could be beneficial to you both?

- If she feels that the way you behave is a contributing factor in her controlling behaviour, you could offer to go to couples counselling. A good counsellor or therapist will listen to both sides of the story and help you work through any joint issues. He or she should be able to help you identify whether each of you is taking responsibility for your own behaviour or trying to blame the other inappropriately.

Explore any underlying issues with your partner. In his book *Love is Never Enough* (1988), the 'founder' of cognitive behaviour therapy, Aaron T. Beck, says that arguments are often not about what they seem to be about – that is, the things a partner does wrong, something he did or didn't do. Often they are about the 'symbolic meanings' partners attach to each other's actions. So, while one person will be laid back about a partner coming home late from work because she went for a drink with a colleague, another might feel this is 'proof' that her partner is disrespectful, uncaring, irresponsible or having an affair.

Understanding what it is that your partner reads into the things you do that makes her angry or upset, and the meaning she attaches to it, could be the basis of better communication between you, as it might get to the very heart of the problem. If you can identify the meanings she attaches to your actions, then you can offer the meanings *you* attach to your actions – they're probably very different from your partner's. For example, for you, going for a drink after work with a colleague might be about taking opportunities to have a laugh, develop friendships, relax or make useful work contacts and has absolutely nothing to do with disrespecting your partner. Trying to 'step into your partner's shoes' to see the situation from her perspective could engender real empathy and understanding between you, which might dissipate the original hurt feelings and/or provide a basis for compromise. You could also try some of the ideas in Chapter 14, which offer ways to deal with unhelpful black and white thinking and a tendency to catastrophize.

How to cope with controlling behaviour

Give up the fight and stop trying to change your partner. Instead, reinvest your energies in your own life and your own interests. This isn't selfish – by doing so you are making your life work better for you as an individual and improving the sustainability of your relationship.

Embrace the idea that no one's life is perfect. If your partner can't or won't change, but you still want to be with her, then it might help to start from the premise that for most people, life is a constant challenge with myriad difficulties to overcome, rather than assume that happiness is a right and always achievable. Seeing the bigger picture of the good, bad and everything in between will help prevent you from focusing only on the problems.

Don't collude with controlling behaviour. By putting in boundaries so that your partner's need to control doesn't govern your life, you may be able to tolerate her behaviour much better. So, take a step back and don't get hooked into going along with things just for a 'quiet life', unless you feel genuinely able to tolerate her behaviour and it doesn't diminish you to do so.

Be guided by what you feel is *reasonable* in any given situation. If it doesn't feel reasonable, don't do it.

If your partner has mild controlling tendencies or her need to control is mostly about her own behaviour – she's not directly trying to control you – it might help if you work at seeing the need to control as being merely a part of her, not the whole person. This may seem like a trivial distinction, but, even in relationships, we can end up categorizing our partners as being one particular type of person and not see the whole picture. Look back at what attracted you to her in the first place. Make a note of all her positive qualities. Her tendency to control may be a dominating daily force in her life and in yours, but is there a way you could focus on other aspects that don't grate on you so much? By shifting your perspective – almost as though you are consciously shifting the 'lens' through which you see her – you may be able to tolerate such behaviour better.

Another idea is to try and 'screen out' the parts you find annoying. If you focus too hard on any annoying habit, then it can become overwhelming. Can you find a way to ignore the annoying bits and tune in more to the aspects of your partner that you like?

If you find certain things about the relationship difficult, try to be open about that. Even if your partner says that she can't stop her controlling behaviour (or refuses to get help in the form of counselling, for instance), she might be able to modify certain aspects. Would she accept your help to try?

Ask for what you need. For example, you might need more privacy, more time on your own, more opportunities to pursue your education, a hobby or your career. All these might enable you to enjoy each other's company more when you are together.

Don't put your life 'on hold' until her problem is sorted out. Make sure that you make the most of any opportunities to enjoy your life as much as you can.

You might want to try the mindfulness exercises on page 106. As we saw in Chapter 9, the art of mindfulness helps you to live more 'moment to moment' rather than in the past or future. If you're living with someone who is very controlling, there might be the tendency to be constantly 'on guard', as you're forever anticipating what she might say or do next. You might also spend time thinking about all the things she's done in the past. Living more in the present may radically reduce both of these patterns of thinking. It can also help you to enjoy the times when her controlling behaviour isn't so prominent. Because you're able to enjoy such moments more, good times are likely to be less overshadowed by anticipating what might come next.

Aim to achieve balance in your life. The more you focus on the negative aspects of living with a controlling partner, the less balanced your life is likely to be. Restore it by taking up new interests, having more fun, having more time to relax, spending more time with your children or whatever helps.

It might be worth looking more closely at why you chose your partner in the first place, particularly if other partners you have had have also been controlling. If you sense that there is a repeat pattern, do you know why you might have chosen someone like this?

Does she remind you of someone else earlier in your life who treated you badly? Perhaps, in a strange way, the pattern of behaviour feels familiar and therefore 'comfortable' because it's what you know. That is not a reason for continuing to accept her behaviour, though.

Perhaps you have low self-esteem and don't think that you deserve any better. This may be reinforced if your partner is controlling in such a way that she puts you down or tells you that you will never find anyone else.

Unravelling the mystery of repeat patterns like these could be something worth talking to a counsellor about.

Ask yourself if you're in what's called a 'codependent' relationship. Codependency is an unhealthy way of relating to others, where both partners tend to have low self-esteem, struggle to set appropriate boundaries and find it difficult to behave as adults. Typically, one person 'takes care' of the other, even if it means not taking care of themselves, so they end up in the role of 'rescuer' or 'martyr', while the other adopts controlling behaviour patterns in a bid to prevent the other abandoning them. Neither of them is capable of sustaining a healthy, adult, intimate relationship.

Counselling can help you identify if you're codependent on each other and there are many books on the topic.

Should I end the relationship?

If the control freak in your life can't or won't change, you might be considering leaving. Finishing a relationship, particularly a long-standing one or where you've invested so much emotionally or have children together is, of course, never easy – even if it's what you want.

So, how can you know the answer to this big question?

Exercise: Should I stay or should I go?

These ten key questions might help you decide.

1. What is my instant gut answer to that question?
2. How do I feel, right now, in this moment, thinking about what's right for me?
3. How will I know when I've had enough?
4. What would need to happen for me to be sure that I should leave?
5. Has it happened yet?
6. Do I want to wait until it has happened?
7. If I stay, would I be staying for the wrong reasons?
8. What would be the main things that I would gain by leaving?
9. What would I advise someone else in my position to do?
10. If I imagine myself in 10 or 15 years' time, looking back at my decision to stay or go, would I be most glad that I'd left or most glad I'd stayed?

It might help to reflect on why you have stayed in the relationship for as long as you have. One possibility is that being in a relationship fraught with conflict can, in a strange but unhelpful way, be very energizing. Somehow you can feel more alive when you are fighting your corner, trying to keep one step ahead of your partner, feeling a victim, battling to be right or putting a lot of energy into trying to get your partner to change. If you took away all of those things from your relationship, ask yourself, 'What would be left?' Would there be happy times? Would you feel truly alive and adequately fulfilled in the relationship or would it feel so empty that it would make you realize you're not happy at all?

If you had the chance, where would you direct the energy you are currently using up to combat your partner's controlling behaviour? What would you do instead that would make you happy – what would make your heart, soul and mind sing?

Another way to help you make this decision is to think about how 'authentic' your life feels to you at the moment. What does that mean? Well, it could mean, for example, when we are being true to ourselves, following our own conscience, doing the right things for the right reasons, living by our own moral code, our own values. It could also mean when we follow a path in life because it feels right, are able to be genuine in relationships and aren't afraid to be ourselves, rather than how someone else wants us to be; that we aren't dependent on other people's approval, are aware of our own limitations and struggles, but still able to move forward in life, living 'authentically'.

Is the relationship you're in a barrier to living authentically? What would living more authentically mean to you? What do you need to do to live more authentically? Could you make that possible in the relationship you are in? If the answer is no, then what does that tell you?

Another factor that needs to be considered when trying to decide if you should stay in a relationship or leave is the effect that living with a controlling partner might be having on your children. The charity Refuge, which offers help for women and children in violent relationships, says that, in nine out of ten incidents, children are in the same or next-door room during a domestic violence incident. It's not known what effects psychological abuse of one partner by another might have on children, but Refuge says that all children living with abuse are under stress and that stress may lead to any of the following:

- bedwetting
- difficulties at school
- withdrawal
- tantrums
- vandalism
- problems in school, such as truancy, difficulties with learning
- attention-seeking behaviour
- nightmares
- insomnia
- anxiety, depression or fear of being abandoned
- feelings of inferiority
- drug or alcohol abuse
- eating disorders
- physical illnesses, such as constant colds, headaches, mouth ulcers, asthma, eczema.

Sometimes it's very difficult for a parent to know how far witnessing controlling behaviour and/or psychological abuse is affecting their children. You can help them by talking with them, helping them to express their feelings, teaching them that abuse of any kind is unacceptable, helping to boost their confidence, praising them and helping them to understand that the abuse is not their fault. You can also help them see that it's OK for them to seek help by setting an example and showing that you are not afraid to seek help for yourself.

One concern might be that you're afraid of what your partner might do if you left. Whether you're a man or a woman, you might be afraid that your partner will be violent towards you. You might fear that your partner will never leave you alone so it would be difficult to start a new relationship. You might be terrified that your partner will take your children from you and refuse to let you see them. You might be afraid of leaving your children with him or her.

These are very real and important concerns and, if you want to leave, it is vital that you find good support from wherever you can – friends, family, the police, a refuge. You may need to find out your rights regarding the family home and custody of the children. In the UK, the Citizens Advice Bureau may be able to advise on this or give you sources of information. The important thing is to be aware of your own and your children's safety, particularly if you are concerned that your partner might become violent or aggressive or you feel afraid.

Refuge, a domestic violence charity, offers practical information about keeping yourself and your children safe if you are being abused (see Useful addresses).

Ultimately, only you can know what is right for you, or you and your child or children. One danger is that you may have become so used to being controlled, so used to living a shadow of a life with someone who never sees your point of view, doesn't value you for who you are or wants things all his own way, that you have come to expect very little. You may even believe the lie that you're not good enough to be with anyone else or live independently on your own without crumbling. Your life may be limited, so you may feel that you don't have the money or the confidence to put the building blocks in place to design a new life for yourself.

If all the hopes and dreams you started out with have been dashed and you're starting from scratch, the journey can seem too difficult even to start, but it is possible. It sounds like a cliché, but there's a Chinese saying that goes like this:

The journey of 1000 miles starts with a single step.

That first step might be a decision. It might be getting support from people who love you, even if at the moment you are estranged from them. It might be about looking back at your life and remembering who you once were and finding that, yes, once you were resilient, once you would have known what to do and been able to do it. That might give you hope or put you back in touch with a sense of your ability to cope. It might be about making a telephone call for help or seeking counselling. It might be about putting your children's welfare above everything else.

By looking deep inside yourself, you may be able to get a sense of what you really need to do and summon up the resources to help you do that, whatever it is.

12

Coping with controlling parents

It's not only partners who can be controlling, as anyone who lives with a controlling parent will know.

Rosie, 28, still lives with her parents because she simply can't afford to move out.

Rosie

My parents have been brilliant in many ways because they supported me through university and, since then, the only job I could get is low-paid, so I can't afford even to rent my own place.

On the whole, we get on well, but arguments erupt because they don't appreciate that I need my own space, I want to go out and come in when it suits me and I want to live as independently as possible, even though we're all under the same roof.

I don't think that my mother realizes she's controlling because she sees it as she's only being helpful. She just doesn't get that, at going on 30, I have a right to live my life the way I want and she shouldn't invade my privacy by going in my room when I'm not there, even if it is trying to be helpful by doing my washing, etc. I once got the third degree because she found a packet of condoms in my bedside drawer, which is ludicrous, given my age!

I'm happy to pull my weight around the house, but she fusses around and won't let me take any responsibility. My tea is on the table when I get home from work, whether I want it or not, and, given that I work shifts, it sometimes means when I get back at 11 p.m.

I find it suffocating at times. I put up with it because I love them and, in any case, I don't really have a choice at the moment.

Statistics show that more and more young people are – by choice or necessity – continuing to live in the family home. In the UK, the Office for National Statistics (ONS), in its annual report on social trends (April 2009), said that almost one third of men and one fifth of women aged between 20 and 34 now live at home with their parents. Other research found that the trend is spreading to older people, with 300,000 people in the 35 to 54 age group living with their parents, too.

The reasons for people choosing to stay at home or being unable to move away in the first place are clear: lack of affordable housing, more people staying on in education, general financial difficulties and, according to one survey, just wanting 'home comforts', are some of the key ones. Let's not forget either that some grown-up children genuinely enjoy living with and get on well with their parents!

You don't have to be living at home to suffer from the effects of controlling parents, of course, but, if you are relying on them financially, then that may make it harder to escape controlling patterns of behaviour. Even if you do live away from your parents, they may still be controlling, in terms of what they expect from you or how you should live your life, in terms of friends and partners or – and this is one of the biggest areas of contention – how you bring up your children.

So, what can you do about it? First, it can be helpful to know what's behind their actions. This will tell you something about their intentions and, in turn, help you to understand how you might best handle them. See if any of the parent types I've suggested below fit your own situation. I've also suggested specific strategies that you could try according to each type.

The classic authoritarian parent

Intention behind behaviour

To be right at all costs.

Profile

This type of parent may have been brought up in exactly the same way that he is trying to parent you.

He will tend to have rigid expectations, strong and 'traditional' values, demand respect regardless of how he behaves and an unerring need to be right. He will find it hard to be flexible, have a 'stiff upper lip' attitude and may find it difficult to show empathy.

He may have low self-esteem and the need to be right could be a cover for having a low opinion of himself. He will often see things as black or white and, to him, backing down may be seen as a threat to his sense of self.

He doesn't see the need to negotiate a compromise so that everyone is happy. The only way is *his* way.

Things you might hear him say

- 'You'll do as I say, or else ...'

- 'I don't care what you think.'
- 'I'm not discussing it.'

Strategies

This is the most difficult type of parent to cope with because he will have the most rigid type of thinking of all the types of parents, but these ideas may help.

- Be specific and firm about what you want or what you're going to do, but match his anger or irritability with a soft, calm voice and quiet certainty. Then he will know that you mean what you say, but you're not prepared to have a slanging match.
- Don't get into debates to try and change your parent's mind. Instead, use the 'scratched record' technique. To do this, narrow down what you want to say to one or two key statements and restate those rather than continue to get drawn into impossible arguments, make new points or retaliate regarding new accusations. Then your message will be clear, concise and consistent.
- Talk to him about his upbringing, what life was like for him when he was younger. People who always have to be right are often quite sad, unfulfilled, angry people whose brusqueness doesn't win them many friends, so invest some time in trying to understand him and offering empathy. It may soften his heart a bit.
- Keep him in the loop about your life. While he may appear to be domineering, controlling and critical of everything you do, he may, deep down, just wish that he were more a part of your life but simply doesn't know how to be any other way. If you can give him opportunities to be a part of your life and meet your friends, and ask his opinion, even if you don't like the answer, you will help keep the lines of communication open and help to create a climate where change for him is at least a little more possible.
- If you simply can't stand it any more, you may feel that a bid for complete independence is the only possible solution. If you do decide to leave or take the more drastic measure of cutting off contact completely, think about the possibility that if you're taking a black and white attitude to your father, then you may effectively be perpetuating the very attitudes you find difficult to tolerate in him.

It's sometimes helpful to remember that, no matter how difficult you're finding things at the moment, you may feel differently in the future. Then, you might be glad that you somehow managed to 'keep the door open' and maintained contact.

The sacrificing parent

Intention behind behaviour

That you shouldn't make the same mistakes she made and she only wants the best for you.

Profile

This type of parent has your best interests at heart and she is determined that she will do all that is in her power to help and advise you. Unfortunately, her passion for helping you may sometimes cross a boundary and become intrusive, particularly if she insists on trying to help and offer advice when you simply don't want it.

Often this happens as a result of her being weighed down by her own failures, fears and disappointments and not trusting you to make your own mistakes and learn from them. Although she has your best interests at heart, the energy she invests in helping or even moulding you, ironically, stops her from hearing what you want. As a result, although she will feel that she is motivated by love and is passionate about wanting the best for you, she will often bulldoze through your life, sure that she 'knows best' and her way is the only way. She wants to save you from yourself, blind to the possibility that, actually, you might want to do things differently.

Essentially, this type of parent is prone to treating you like a child.

Things you might hear her say

- 'I only want the best for you.'
- 'I'm going to give you advice whether you want it or not.'
- 'Trust me, I know best.'

Strategies

This type of parent is more likely than most to listen to reason and may be willing to change her behaviour if you can explain how it really makes you feel. She will probably have some awareness of what she's doing, but doesn't know *how* to change. Here are some ideas that you might like to try.

- Make a date to talk to her about 'something important'. Ensure that it's a time when you can sit down together in a period of relative calm, when there are no major contentious issues already being debated.
- Start by emphasizing that you understand she only has your best interests at heart and give one or two examples of times when you've been specially aware of this and how it has made you feel good and/or been very valuable to you.

- Begin to explain to her how you're feeling about the way she treats you and give examples. Be careful to own your own stuff and start with 'I' sentences. So, for example, say, 'I feel sad because I feel I have to do things the way you want me to' or 'I feel powerless sometimes because I feel you help me so much that I'm not learning to be independent; I think I need to make my own mistakes and begin to learn from them'. These kinds of 'I' statements will have more impact than an accusatory 'You make me feel really annoyed when you interfere in my room' or 'You need to butt out of my life', which is more likely to put her on the defensive and end up in an argument.
- Ask for what you want – and be specific. What specific things would you like her to stop doing? Explain why that is.
- Explain, too, how all this could change your relationship with her for the better. For example, would you feel more able to talk to her or ask her advice (whereas at the moment you might tend to avoid her or avoid asking for advice because you'll get it whether you like it or not)? Would it help make your relationship closer?
- Anticipate her fears about relinquishing control. Ask how you can help her. For example, she may fear that if she backs off from helping you, that you'll be less dependent on her and therefore there'll be less contact with you overall. You might be able to bridge the gap by promising to phone regularly or meet up regularly for a meal.
- Consider that a compromise may be a good starting point.

The self-serving parent

Intention behind behaviour

That he only wants the best for you because it's the best for him.

Profile

This type of parent may be overly worried about his reputation or image, so his need to control you may be rooted in wanting to keep up appearances, impress family, friends or even neighbours. He will like to do 'the right thing' in terms of cultural or traditional expectations, which for him may be linked with class or religion.

Often his expectations are totally out of kilter with what might reasonably be expected. His language is black and white, itself a barrier to real communication because you're having to fight overly dramatic viewpoints and stereotypes from the start. He also tends to catastrophize about small mistakes or his perceptions of the consequences of your actions and may be liberal with name-calling and criticism.

Things you might hear him say

- 'I'll never be able to hold my head up in this street again.'
- 'What will the family think?'
- 'You're no daughter/son of mine if you behave like that.'

Strategies

Entrenched attitudes like this are hard to break through and effecting major change may be very difficult or impossible, but the following might help.

- Chances are that the main areas of disagreement between you occur regularly and are often similar in content – to do with jobs, partners, leisure-time activities, personal habits, attitudes. Getting into debates to try and change his mind may be futile, unless he will be won over by cleverly argued analytical points. Instead, use the 'scratched record' technique, mentioned earlier.
- One difficulty with this type of parent is that he may find it hard to see you as an individual, because his view of you is tied up with cultural expectations. Talking to him about his own childhood and family life may help. Did conforming make him happy? Were his own parents happy? Were his siblings happy? What were the differences between his family members? Do all family members need to be the same and conform in order to be accepted? Can difference be celebrated within families?
- Quietly muster support from people you know your father respects within the family in order to help your case.

This last strategy is risky, as he will value 'keeping face' and might see talking outside the immediate family as a loss of face in itself, almost a kind of betrayal. If, though, you sense that he might listen to a close relative you know is sympathetic to your plight, this strategy could be a useful one. If this can be done sensitively, it will protect him from losing face, which, in turn, will make the possibility of change a little more likely.

The martyr parent

Intention behind behaviour

To keep you hooked in to her needs so you never leave her.

Profile

This type of parent is self-serving and hungry for your attention, your love or your care and will stop at nothing to get it.

A typical martyr parent is a master of manipulating her children to get what she wants. Her mission is to stay needy, or appear needy, so that you can never leave her – if physically, at least not emotionally.

She will make you feel guilty (subtly if necessary), plead or cry in order to get what she wants. She may be careful to be not overtly demanding, but the tone of her voice or even her body language leaves you under no illusion as to what is expected of you.

A martyr parent will present herself as a victim, whether she realizes it or not, even if she often says, 'Oh, don't worry about me.' Whatever words are used, you can end up feeling controlled because the true message ('don't leave me') is as large, obvious and unmistakable as an elephant sitting in your living room.

It's important to say here that some parents are genuinely needy. They may have disabilities, be ill, may have psychological problems or be vulnerable and so trying to keep you close to them may be a matter of survival, and so they may be very afraid of losing you. In such situations, it's easy to label a person a 'martyr', when in fact he or she is genuinely vulnerable.

Sorting out in your own mind what is 'reasonable' will help, but it may never be enough to fulfil her needs. That, though, is her problem, not yours.

Things you might hear her say

- 'Oh I'll be fine, stuck here on my own. You go out if you really want to ...'
- 'I could never manage without you.'
- 'You'd do more for me if you loved me.'

Strategies

- Decide on the boundaries that need to be drawn between you and your parent and stick to them rigidly. In the past, you may have been wishy-washy about boundaries – for example, giving in to her demands on some occasions, albeit for understandable reasons – but this may have fuelled her expectations and made the situation even more intractable.
- Look at your own motivation. If you frequently change your plans because your parent asks you to, either overtly or obliquely, why do you change them? Maybe there are good reasons. If your mother is ill and genuinely needs your help or can't be left and no one else can help, that might be a very legitimate reason. If, however, you stay only because you're fed up with the arguments, you don't have the confidence or nerve to say no, because you feel guilty if you go out or because your mother will make your life hell when you get back, then they're all less sound reasons.

You might find it helpful to do some work on yourself and explore your own motivations about what keeps you stuck in such an unhealthy relationship. Think about the changes you'd like to make.

- Explore other options if there are other family members who could help and take the pressure off you. There's no point starting with a hoped-for outcome, though, as if they don't deliver for whatever reason, then you may feel disappointed and resentful. You can't force other people to help. It might seem unfair and unjust, but if you keep a mental tally of who's doing what and the rights and wrongs of that, you'll always be unhappy. Narrow it down and focus on whether or not *you* feel happy with the amount and quality of what *you're* doing. That's all that counts. Let others take responsibility for their own decisions.

- In some situations, you may need to be cruel to be kind. Saying no may seem cruel, but you deserve to have a life too and live your life your own way.

The empty nester

Intention behind behaviour

To put off the day you leave home for as long as possible.

Profile

An empty nester is easy to identify. In short, he loves you and doesn't want you to leave home!

He fears that you'll go off into the big wide world and leave him, and he can't bear to let you go. What's more, time-wise, your leaving may herald the start of middle age for him – and he's going kicking and screaming all the way!

Things you might hear him say

- 'I'm going to miss you so much when you leave.'
- 'I want you to write home and phone me every day.'
- 'We've decided to move to be nearer your place!'

Strategies

A parent who is controlling because he is dreading you leaving home is, in many ways, the easiest to deal with; a bit of common sense and a lot of empathy is all that's required.

- Talk to him about how he feels about you leaving. Don't leave this to the last minute. Even if he hasn't voiced his fears about you leaving, he might be coaxed to talk to you about it, if you'll listen.

- Ask him if he has any particular fears about you leaving, so you know the kinds of strategies that might help him to feel better – keeping in touch regularly and so on.
- Don't lose sight of your own sense of what's reasonable and what's not. Don't be tempted to stray over that line to appease them. If he's asking too much of you, negotiate down. If you can do this in a spirit of caring for him, and offering a reasonable alternative that shows you care, then this might be all that's required to ease his anxiety and reduce his controlling behaviour.
- Remember, it's often the small things that count – the texts for no reason, a thoughtful gift when you go home for the weekend, sending a postcard unexpectedly just to show you care, asking his advice occasionally, making him feel wanted and useful. This is one time when turning up with a bag of dirty washing can be a true kindness rather than exploitation!

The 'I dreamed a dream' parent

Intention behind behaviour

That you live out her unfulfilled dreams, whether you want to or not.

Profile

This type of parent is a bit like the sacrificing parent above, but the big difference here is that for the 'I dreamed a dream' parent, none of what she does for you is in any way 'a sacrifice' for her because she's living her life through you. Your life is, largely, her life, with not enough degrees of separation between you.

Such a parent will convince herself that you want the kind of life she wishes she could have had for herself. She is a master of convincing herself and others that what she's doing 'for you' is what you want, when it's really what she wants for herself, by proxy. She may even openly admit this. It may be that she had an unhappy childhood, or tried to achieve a particular dream and failed, so is determined that your life will be full and exciting.

Maybe this sounds good, but as a child you might have been rushed between different activities or shoe-horned into one special activity that your mother was sure you'd excel at, but you never really enjoyed. Some 'pushy parents' who insist that their children should take time off school and put all their free time into activities such as modelling, appearing in TV adverts, ice-skating, gymnastics, acting, swimming and so on with a view to fame, fortune or sporting excellence can fall into this category.

You may have learned early on that agreeing to whatever your mother lined up for you was a way of being loved and making her happy. So, if asked, 'You do want to do this, don't you?' you might have said 'Yes', especially if you were made aware that your mother was making financial sacrifices for you, even if truthfully you hated it or would have preferred to spend more time with your friends or do a range of other more ordinary activities. As an older teenager or young adult, your mother may still have been trying to encourage you to choose certain jobs and partners you don't feel were right for you.

Things you might hear her say

- 'It would make me so proud if you ...'
- 'I'm not pushing you into this, am I ...?
- 'If you do this it would make up for the time when ...'

Strategies

This kind of parent may have less self-awareness than some others, so could find it harder to see your point of view or may just discount it. Setting firm boundaries and knowing what you really want can be particularly difficult for you. You may have become so used to fulfilling her needs that you've never actually discovered what *you* want or are capable of.

- Knowing what you want or, at the very least, what you *don't* want is a key starting point. The more confidence you have about this, the greater your sense of self and the more you'll be able to put it across with conviction. It might be useful to do some research. If career is the issue, you might consider career counselling to see what types of work you might be suited to, for example.
- Improve your assertiveness skills and take every opportunity to practise them in non-stressful situations outside your immediate family environment, where it's not the end of the world if you don't 'win' the point. Act 'as if' you are assertive. Say the sorts of things you imagine an assertive person might say and use everyday situations to hone your skills. In other words, broaden your experience of hearing yourself say 'no', 'I don't want that', 'I don't want to do that', 'I'd rather do this', 'I don't agree with you' and so on. If you make the effort to practise, you will improve and your anxiety levels should begin to drop.
- Use your assertiveness skills with your mother, remembering that being assertive is not the same as being aggressive. Ask for what you want, say no to things you don't want. Be consistent so your mother eventually grasps the idea that if she just keeps trying to persuade you, you're not eventually going to give in.

The mixed-up parent

Intention behind behaviour

To get the love, devotion and respect that he doesn't get from his partner from you instead.

Profile

This type of parent has a rather skewed notion of what parenthood is. His boundaries may be sketchy, and so he will work hard at being seen to be your 'best friend' rather than your parent. Of course, it's great to have a parent who is also a great friend, but where this stems from not having a partner of his own or not getting what he needs from his own relationship, then he can become demanding and controlling in an unhealthy way.

Things you might hear him say

- 'Don't you love me any more?'
- 'If you really loved me, you wouldn't do that/you'd do this.'
- 'Are you going to meet your friends/go to a club? I'll just get my jacket ...'

Strategies

It can be hard to extricate yourself from this type of relationship, but firm boundaries and consistency will help, along with an awareness of the kind of relationship you're aiming for instead.

- Think about what is and what isn't acceptable in your relationship, so you are clear about what boundaries you need to set.
- Improve your assertiveness skills (see above).
- Say clearly what you're prepared to do and what you're not prepared to do.
- Encourage your father to broaden his own life if you feel that he is too wrapped up in you.

Living with controlling parents is never easy. Chances are they're doing their best with the resources they have. They may have slipped into patterns of behaviour that you find unacceptable but they've just got used to. Maybe the way forward is gentle negotiation or learning to increase your tolerance threshold, or a mixture of both. It will certainly help if you can both work at seeing each other as fallible human beings who mostly try their best and who inevitably make mistakes along the way. Good luck!

13

Control freaks at work – and how to survive them

The workplace control freak is often the sort of person most people would describe as a 'bully'.

The late Tim Field, author of the worldwide bestselling book *Bully in Sight* (1996) and founder of the UK National Workplace Bullying Advice Line (now known as Bully OnLine.org) estimated that 1 person in 30 is a serial bully. He defined workplace bullying as:

> persistent unwelcome behaviour, mostly using unwarranted or invalid criticism, nit-picking, fault-finding, also exclusion, isolation, being singled out and treated differently, being shouted at, humiliated, excessive monitoring, having verbal and written warnings imposed, and much more. In the workplace, bullying usually focuses on distorted or fabricated allegations of underperformance.

Field suggested that the main reason for bullies acting the way that they do is to hide their inadequacy. Though they may be full of hatred and anger, they often have low self-esteem and feel insecure, the bullying serving as a mask for their own poor self-image.

Bullies tend to target people who are either more popular or competent than they are and/or have a weakness that can be exploited, such as a disability, a different sexual orientation, age or youth, or who would find it hard to get another job for some reason or are psychologically vulnerable in some way – someone who is already anxious, for example. Or there may be no specific reason at all.

Joy, 55, worked in a small finance company. She had been with the company for over 15 years and enjoyed her job – until there was an organizational change and she found herself with a new boss, 20 years younger than her.

Joy
I knew people who had worked with Sheena in the past and didn't like her, but when she was put in charge of the small team I was part of, it was me she targeted. I think it was partly because I had been there longer than anyone else, so maybe she saw me as a threat.

From the start, she gave me unrealistic deadlines I couldn't possibly meet, she harassed me to finish work and then didn't look at it, she criticized me in front of others, she was sarcastic and rude. I felt she was constantly watching my every move and hoping I'd make mistakes, and I found it very wearing and stressful. She asked me several times if I'd thought of taking early retirement, making it clear she wanted me to leave.

She was infuriating to work for because on the occasions I did need more direction, she would be evasive. I think she wanted me to look foolish or turn in poor work.

In the end, I decided to leave. I couldn't really afford to give up work, but I couldn't stand it. My mum had left me some money in her will, so I gave in my notice.

People have said to me I should have made a formal complaint, but I knew I would have had to keep notes about all the things she said and did and I just couldn't face it. She was a bully and unfortunately I let her win, but at least I don't have to put up with it any more.

Joy's story illustrates well how much power and control a bully in the workplace can wield. The National Bullying Helpline (see Useful addresses) suggests that 80 per cent of managers know that bullying occurs in their workplace. In Britain alone, it costs the economy £3.7 billion annually due to the victims of bullying taking time off because of stress, the cost of dispute resolution and compensation payments.

The 'National Workplace Bullying Survey 2005' was one of the UK's biggest ever investigations into workplace bullying conducted by Digital Opinion and commissioned by *Personnel Today* magazine and the Andrea Adams Trust, a charity helping those bullied in the workplace. Over 30,000 human resources professionals were invited to take part, of which 1391 responded. Just over half of these said that they had been bullied at work. The respondents cited a variety of bullying behaviours, with unfair criticism, intimidating behaviour and humiliation/ridicule being the most common. The effects on the victims included a lowering of confidence and self-esteem and worrying about going to work. Over 43 per cent said that it had affected the quality of their work and 17 per cent said it had caused them to take time off.

It's worth bearing in mind that there are no easy answers to bullying in the workplace, but there are things you can do. Talking to others about what's happening may help to empower you in such a way that you no longer feel so vulnerable to a bully, or give you confidence to seek further help. Certainly it seems sensible to go about whatever action you do decide to take in a considered way, after taking advice.

What to do about a workplace control freak

An action plan

- If you feel that you are being bullied, consider standing up for yourself on each and every occasion you can. This is a hugely daunting task if you don't feel confident, the bully is in a more senior position than you or you're afraid it will worsen the situation. If the bully realizes that you never stand up for yourself, she will have no incentive to stop what she is doing. By contrast, if you can muster some courage to stand up for yourself, each time, even if it is in small ways, then she may stop. Doing so will be important if you make a complaint or, indeed, if the bully makes a complaint about you or unsubstantiated allegations about the standard of your work.

- Find out if your place of work has an antibullying or harassment policy and ask for a copy. According to the Andrea Adams Trust, around 60 per cent of UK companies should have such a policy. If you are a member of a union, it may be able to offer you support and advice. Find out if there is a formal complaints system for you to complain about the behaviour of the bully. The National Bullying Helpline delivers specialist training for employers, with comprehensive dispute resolution training, investigations into bullying and mediation services, as well as a helpline for employees who would like advice about bullying (see Useful addresses). It's important to get help and advice at an early stage.

- Don't isolate yourself. Remember the bullying is *not* your fault, so get support from coworkers who can see what is going on, if they're willing to do so.

- Keep a diary of any bullying behaviour you experience, as you may need it if you, or someone else, makes a formal complaint. Include the day, date, time and place and what was said. As far as possible, record the exact words used, your response and how you felt at the time of the incident. It may be able to be shown that you politely told the bully you were unhappy with what was said to you or how it was said, or that you told the bully you thought her actions were unreasonable in some way, but then she continued to do the same thing on a number of occasions. In this way, if your complaint is taken up, allegations are made about you, or you find yourself with a written warning for something the bully says you have or have not done, you will have more ammunition than if you said nothing or can only be vague about what happened when and so on.

- On a practical level, it is best to avoid being alone with the bully, where possible. If you have your own office, leave the door open if the bully is with you. If she closes the door, find a reason to get up and open the door and say that you want the door left open.

- If the bullying takes place in front of others, speak to them afterwards about it. Find out what they think they saw and heard and keep a note of what they said, or ask directly for their support.
- Keep a note of any days you have taken off sick due to stress. It's advisable to talk to your doctor about what's happening to you at work and request counselling if you feel it might be helpful to talk to someone about it.

How to speak up for yourself

You don't have to be clever with words or make a speech. Even one, short, to-the-point sentence to make your views known is better than saying nothing at all. It may sound silly, but practise some of the lines you could say in private, maybe in front of a mirror, and in a confident voice.

You probably know the bully well enough to have worked out how she operates and what kinds of things she does or says to you. Bullies, though, are masters of finding new ways to bully people, so it's difficult to prepare for every situation. Don't worry about 'fluffing your lines'. It's still better to say something 'badly' or awkwardly than it is not to stand up for yourself.

Don't worry about blushing, stumbling, having a wobbly voice, forgetting what you want to say or getting it wrong. What matters is that you're showing the bully you won't just let her walk all over you. Even if you think you've made a mess of it in some way, she will get the underlying message that you're not prepared to put up with it. Hopefully, the more you give it a try, the more confident you will become, which will boost your self-esteem.

What sorts of things could you say? Here, it can be helpful to stick to how *you* feel rather than make accusations. Once you've said what you have to say, don't be drawn into further discussion, argument or justifying what you've said. You don't have to answer any of the bully's questions. Knowing this can be liberating. Empower yourself, not the bully.

Remember, too, that it's OK to ask for what you want. It sounds obvious, but often we don't do it. Also, repeat your original statement. This keeps it simple and will reduce the pressure on you, especially if you feel that you won't know how to respond to what the bully says next. It will also throw the bully off balance if you refuse to engage further with her and it will make your original statement more powerful, more memorable. If you don't do this and get drawn into explaining, justifying or amplifying on what you've said, there's a danger that your original message will be watered down in some way, or twisted by the bully.

Here are some examples of the kinds of things that you could say. Adapt them to your own particular circumstance and the way you'd normally speak.

- 'I don't accept your constant criticisms of me.'
- 'I want you to know that being on the receiving end of your constant criticisms/allegations is making me feel anxious/hurt/upset/stressed.'
- 'I feel intimidated when you shout/bang things down on my desk/invade my personal space/humiliate me in front of others. I want you to know that I find your behaviour totally unacceptable and unnecessary. I want you to stop.'
- 'I don't like the way you speak sarcastically to me/put me down in front of my colleagues/criticize me in meetings and I want you to stop.'
- 'I find your behaviour towards me unreasonable and unacceptable, in particular because you are setting me unachievable targets/you are constantly criticizing me/you frequently make unsubstantiated allegations against me/you put me down too often/you make fun of me/you make fun of me in front of colleagues/you undermine me in front of colleagues and I want you to stop these actions or I will take further advice.'
- 'I want to tell you formally that I feel your recent treatment of me has been unreasonable and I want you to stop.'

Being on the receiving end of bullying is not just deeply unpleasant, it can also lead to anxiety, depression and stress-related illness. It can be so unbearable that some people feel driven to suicide.

You are not alone. There is support out there for you and seeking help is one step you can take to empower yourself. You can find further information from sources listed in the Useful addresses section.

14

Self-help for control freaks

You may be reading this book because other people have remarked that you're a control freak, or because you recognize that this particular label fits you and you want to do something about it.

I hope that the information given throughout the book has been of help (for example, did any of the types of control freak described in Chapters 3 to 7 seem to be a 'fit' for you?) You might want to consider counselling, which could help you to explore what you have learned further. Also, take a look at the following questions, thoughts and self-help suggestions as they might be useful to you.

Do you really want to change?

- Do you accept and believe that your life would be better if you were able to make changes and be less controlling? Would you be willing to try and make changes? If you were successful in making those changes, how would your life be different?
- How would the lives of those around you be different? Would they be happier? How would that affect you? Would you be glad or would you find that threatening in some way?
- If you were less controlling, would you be happier, more relaxed, proud of yourself and more able to make the most of opportunities that come your way?

How controlling are you?

- It might help to think about the ways in which you are controlling or how others experience you controlling them or others. If you're honest, do you feel, deep down, that the way you are behaving is really how you want to be? Is it how you really want to be in your relationships?
- It's important to also know in what ways you *aren't* controlling so that you come to a balanced view of yourself. It might help to take a sheet of paper and make a list of all the aspects of your personality that you like or are proud of. What do you value about yourself?

93

You could also make a list of the behaviours that you want to change.

- How is your behaviour really affecting the people around you, the people you love? Is it making them miserable? Is it affecting their self-esteem or confidence? Does being controlling make you feel good at someone else's expense? How does that make you feel to know that?
- How controlling do you think you are? If 0 is 'not at all controlling' and 10 is 'very controlling', where are you on the scale? How happy are you to be like that? If 0 is 'not happy' and 10 is 'very happy', where are you on the scale? What do those results tell you?

Understanding yourself better

What are the main faulty thought patterns you have that tend to lead to your controlling behaviour?

Do you think in black and white terms? Do you have an 'all or nothing' approach to things? Do you tend to catastrophize when things don't go your way or people in your life make small mistakes? Would learning to give and take a bit more, allowing yourself to be more flexible, make your relationships worse or better?

What long-held views and assumptions do you have that seem to drive your need to be controlling? For example, 'a woman's place is in the home', 'the man should be the breadwinner', 'children should be seen and not heard'. Where do these views and assumptions come from?

Thinking about what your life is like at the moment, and how your views influence your behaviour or affect the people you live with, how helpful or unhelpful is it to hold these views? What does it achieve? Are there any disadvantages to holding these views? What are they? How might life be different if you held different views? Would you be happier? Would the people around you be happier? Even if you feel you can't change your views, how useful would it be to be able to accept that it's OK for other people to have very different views from yours? Do you find the idea that others can hold different views and opinions from you challenging? Why do you think you feel like that?

It might help to think about why you developed a controlling behaviour pattern in the first place. Did something happen in your early life that you feel could be connected to this?

Were you ever abandoned in some way or did you ever *feel* abandoned? Did you suffer a bereavement or other type of loss when you were young that perhaps you couldn't express your feelings about at the time? Was one of your parents an alcoholic? Were you abused? Have you felt let down in your life, particularly by your parents or your partner? Are you repeating as an adult the kind of behaviour you witnessed or were subjected to as you were growing up?

Alternatively, perhaps you're so intent on *not* being the same as your parents that in some way you've gone to the other extreme. If everything was chaotic when you were a child, maybe your need for order and control is somehow connected to that.

Maybe it's none of these and you have your own ideas and theories. What do you think it's about? If you're aware that you are holding on to old patterns of behaviour, they might have been helpful once, but are they still helpful? Are they, instead, ruining your life and the lives of those around you?

What are your fears about changing your views or changing your controlling behaviour? What's the worst that could happen? What would be the benefits? What fears do you have about changing?

Think of someone in your life, past or present, someone you really love and respect. If that person had exactly the same problems as you and you could see it was badly affecting his or her life and the lives of the person's partner and family, what would you advise that person to do?

Tips and techniques

Make a start today

What one, small, achievable change could you make today that might nudge you up that scale a little towards being less controlling? Ask someone close to you what you could change to make the biggest difference.

Banish black and white thinking

People who are very controlling often think in black and white terms. People, places, things, experiences and so on are either at one end of the scale ('amazing, wonderful, brilliant') or at the other ('useless, clueless, pathetic'), with very little grey in between.

This type of faulty thinking is highly damaging because it can lead to extreme thoughts and actions, a tendency to believe you're right over everyone else and getting angry when things go wrong.

What can you do to change this?

Use 'scaling'

When you find yourself thinking that something is a 'total disaster' or something 'must' be done a certain way, use a scale of 0 to 10 to help you reframe that thought. Let's use a simple example so that you can see what I mean.

You like to be punctual and you're due to go out for dinner with your girlfriend. She phones to say that she's running late. Your attitude is that it's a 'total disaster'.

Think of the scale. If 0 is 'not at all a problem' and 10 is a 'total disaster', does the situation really warrant a 10? Is somewhere in between 0 and 10 more appropriate, realistic, helpful?

Ask 'What do I have to lose?'

Are you worried about losing face if you take a more measured attitude or tone – not being 'right', looking 'stupid', looking 'small', or having to back down?

Does sticking to an extreme view make you feel powerful in some way? Does it seem to you to be a good way to live your life and make lasting relationships?

Stop catastrophizing

Have you got into the habit of making a drama out of a crisis or even making a drama out of nothing much at all?

If you're prone to catastrophizing, you may lurch from drama to disaster because you've lost your ability to get things into perspective. This can seem like an exciting way to live. You can go around shouting and swearing, slamming doors and feeling righteous, but what are you missing out on when you're doing all of that? What's it like for the people around you?

Try using the 'scaling' technique described above to help you kick the habit. If it's 'a disaster' that your dinner's not on the table or you've forgotten to iron a blouse, what are you going to be like if a *real* disaster comes your way?

Avoid making automatic negative assumptions about people

- Give people a chance before you make judgements about them.
- Be aware of your prejudices and how they stop you from seeing people as individuals.

Stop trains of automatic negative or unhelpful thoughts

The first task is to learn to recognize that you're having an unhelpful thought in the first place. This sounds obvious, but it's actually very hard to be 'aware' you're having an unhelpful thought before that first thought leads to further unhelpful thoughts, actions or words.

One really good way to become aware of these thoughts very early on is to practise 'mindfulness' (I discussed this earlier, but see the section on pages 106–9 for more about this).

Once you're aware of an unhelpful thought, there are lots of strategies that you can use to help you overcome it. Then you won't resort to old patterns of controlling behaviour, such as criticizing or putting others down, checking up on them, telling them what to do or how to do it, becoming angry and so on. The following ideas should help.

- **Tell yourself 'it's only a thought'** when a thought comes into your mind that you know might be a trigger for your controlling behaviour. The golden rule is to know that *just because you have a thought doesn't mean it's true*. It's just a thought, not necessarily a fact. So, if you suddenly find yourself thinking, 'She's late home from work. She must be seeing someone else', or whatever it is, then remind yourself 'It's just a thought, it's not necessarily true'. Remembering to do this one tiny thing can be very liberating and stop you getting tangled up in unhelpful downward spirals.
- **Distract yourself** by immediately doing something different. For example, you might stand up and leave the room, go into the garden, have a cup of coffee, busy yourself with chores, read a book, watch a DVD or do something physical – running, dancing, gardening, weight training. Distraction is a particularly good 'first aid' strategy, useful in an emergency, such as in situations where you know that, if you don't check yourself, you might end up having a blazing row, alienating others or resorting to name-calling.
- **Question and reframe your thoughts** Some good questions to ask yourself are: 'What's the real evidence for this thought?', 'What other explanations could there be?', 'How many times in the past have I had this or a similar thought and how many of those times have I been wrong?', 'What would happen if I didn't react to this thought and just let it go?', 'What am I really afraid of?' See the following exercise.

Exercise: For and against

If you tend to have the same thought frequently (for example 'he's being unfaithful'), take a sheet of paper and draw a line down the middle. On one side, write down all the 'evidence' *against* the thought or belief being true and, on the other side, write down all the possible alternative explanations you can think of *for* whatever it was that made you have the thought in the first place. Here's an example.

Thought: Partner is having an affair because she's late home again

Evidence against	*Alternative explanations*
• She's never had an affair before as far as I know.	• She forgot the time.
• Really, I don't think she's the kind of person who would do that to me.	• She got carried away enjoying herself and talking to her friends.
• She's always late anyway, so it's not unusual.	• She missed the bus/train again.
• I don't know anything for sure.	• She got caught in traffic.
• I'm always trying to catch her out but I never have yet.	• Maybe she's just taking her time.
• She says she loves me and she wouldn't do anything to hurt me.	• She could be staying at a mate's.
• My family and friends trust her and think I might be overreacting.	• She probably called at her mum's.

Improve your ability to tolerate not knowing

When it comes to controlling behaviour, lots of downward spirals of negative thoughts are partly the result of not being able to tolerate not knowing something for sure.

Make a pact with yourself to endure not knowing more often, without reacting. You will improve your tolerance levels and that will enable you to build up trust of others. If you learn to tolerate not knowing, you are less likely to react in a destructive way in your relationships.

Reduce your levels of stress

• **Remember to breathe!** This sounds crazy but, in difficult moments, we often breathe shallowly, which creates tension in the body and makes clear thinking more difficult. Taking a few slow, long, deep breaths can give you, literally, a 'breathing space' – a moment to pause and reflect before wading in.

- **Set aside times to relax** Relaxing properly can help reduce anxiety and make you feel good. It's good to pamper yourself from time to time. It can help, too, to do things for other people – listen to their problems, try to help, maybe carry out the odd random act of kindness for no reason at all other than it will feel good for them and for you. All these things will help improve your resilience to difficulties.

- **Improve your sleep patterns** If you don't get a good night's sleep, it can increase your levels of stress and irritability. There are plenty of books on sleep, including *Overcoming Insomnia: How to sleep like a dream* by Susan Elliot-Wright (Sheldon Press, 2008).

Improve your resilience

People who are 'resilient' are better able to manage difficult feelings and thoughts, cope with stressful situations, adapt better to change and come to terms with difficulties or even trauma more easily. In short, resilience helps you to tolerate difficulties better so that you are less likely to overreact, sink into depression or practise unhelpful behaviours. We can all improve our levels of resilience. How? Here's how.

- **Think back to times when you know you were more resilient** Think about times when you did do the right thing, coped well and were able to show self-restraint or see the bigger picture.

- **Take regular exercise** as it will give you an outlet for pent-up feelings and increase the 'feel good' hormones (called endorphins) in the body. Walking and running are obvious choices. You might want to consider something like t'ai chi, which is quite difficult to learn but very rewarding and very good for de-stressing. Another benefit is that it helps you to recognize the benefits of embracing both yin and yang. The more controlling you are, the more yang you are, so it is good to discover your yin side, too! Martial arts generally are excellent for helping you to harness your power and control in a safe way.

- **Eat a balanced diet** as eating well can help improve your mood. Eating too much junk food can adversely affect your mood. You can find out more about food and mental health by visiting Mind's website (<www.mind.org.uk>).

Set yourself goals

If you're really keen to make changes, it might be helpful to set yourself a series of goals. Here are some guidelines.

- **Ensure the goals are realistic and achievable** You might need to break a goal down into smaller, more manageable, steps. Remember, if you try and fail, you can try again.

- **Ask yourself 'the miracle question'** The miracle question orig-inated in solution-focused therapy and I've adapted it for you here. Ask yourself the following series of questions, pausing to answer each one before moving on to the next:
  - If a miracle happened tonight while I was asleep and I woke up tomorrow and didn't feel the need to be controlling any more, what would be different?
  - What would be the first thing I'd notice that would tell me that a miracle had taken place?
  - How else would I know?
  - What else would I notice?

- It's often the smallest details that come in the answers to these ques-tions that provide valuable clues as to what small changes you might be able to make to help you move forward. For example, the first thing you might notice is that you slept well, then that your partner is smiling and warm towards you, then that you feel more relaxed and laid-back, maybe a bit more like your old self. Imagining all this in your mind's eye is a good exercise, as it will give you a glimpse of how your life could be if you were less controlling. It also helps you rehearse and envision a different way of being, which can make the transition to a different way of behaving seem more achievable.

- **Consider keeping a daily diary** where you record your feelings and thoughts, any attempts you made to change, how successful they were and what you might do differently next time. Writing things down like this could help you become more aware, so you notice more about yourself and your patterns of behaviour. You will then be better able to stand back at crucial moments and maybe make different choices about how you relate to others.

Improve your self-esteem and confidence

What are you good at? What skills do you have? What are you proud of? What positive qualities do you have?

Do you find it hard to answer those questions, or find that they are 'I don't know' or 'Nothing'? On a scale of 0 to 10, if 0 is 'very low self-esteem' and 10 is 'very high self-esteem', how do you rate yourself?

If you could improve your self-esteem and confidence, you might have less need to control others. How could you improve your self-esteem? There are many excellent books about improving your self-esteem. I particularly like *Overcoming Low Self-esteem* by Melanie Fennell (2009).

You could also try the following:

- improve your mastery of something you enjoy doing, whether it's singing, playing the guitar, a sport, DIY, a craft, hobby;
- learn a new skill from scratch at an evening class;
- improve your social and communication skills;
- judge yourself less;
- praise yourself more when you put in effort;
- allow yourself to make mistakes without beating yourself up;
- identify core beliefs that dent your self-esteem, such as 'I must always be perfect' (impossible, nobody's always perfect, so, if you hold this core belief, you're bound to feel bad if you fall short of perfection);
- ask for positive feedback from others when you think you deserve it;
- act 'as if' you feel more confident, as this gives you a safe opportunity to try things out and give things a go, and builds your experience of new situations.

Learn to deal better with your anger

Anger can be a healthy emotion and appropriate in some situations. It's what you do with it that's key.

If you can express your feelings without being aggressive, it can help to reduce your anger and may resolve the situation. Unhealthy, unexpressed anger, however, can drive controlling behaviour, while openly expressed anger can spill over into aggression.

You can learn to deal better with anger when things don't go your way.

- Identify what triggers your anger. Is it because people won't do what you want them to do or won't do it in the way you want them to? Is it because you have devised for yourself a set of rules that you've decided need to be stuck to so people who 'disobey' your rules make you angry? If anger is inappropriate or disproportionate to the triggering event, or leads to abuse of others or physical or verbal violence, it makes sense to do something about it.
- How early on do you recognize that you are feeling angry? Does it start suddenly or burn quite slowly or subtly over a period of time?
- Learn to tune in to the early warning signs. They are often physical sensations, such as feeling tight in the chest or stomach, so you can begin to recognize your pattern of anger early on and take action so it doesn't erupt into a situation that you might later regret.

- As soon as you recognize that you are beginning to feel angry, pause for a moment and be aware of your breathing. Chances are you are breathing shallowly. Make a conscious effort to breathe slowly and deeply, as this will reduce tension in the body.
- Pre-prepare a simple mantra – a phrase you remember to repeat to yourself a few times in the early stages of feeling angry. Something like, 'Quit now'.
- Take a five- to ten-minute time out. Remove yourself to a different room or the garden to cool off. Five minutes out of the situation might help you to gather your thoughts and then you can decide to back off or rethink your approach.
- Ask yourself, 'What's the worst that could happen if I were to carry on expressing my anger?' and 'What's the worst that could happen if I were to take a step back from this right now?' Which is the better option?
- Imagine yourself responding in a non-controlling, calm way – almost like rehearsing it in your head. Take a few moments to imagine a scene where normally you might be overly controlling or reacting angrily, which might lead to controlling behaviour. Imagine the whole scene in your mind's eye, but see yourself reacting as you wish you could react. For example, if you get jealous of your partner and might normally quiz her when she gets home about who she's seen, what they talked about and so on, imagine yourself instead just asking her if she's had a good time and giving her a hug. This may sound strange, but if you've imagined a better way to react in your mind's eye, then when you come to act that way, it will feel more familiar and might be easier to do in reality.

Stop trying to be perfect

Are you living your life according to a 'be perfect' script? Does your controlling behaviour, whatever it is, stem from you being a perfectionist? Where did that idea come from? What's your fear of not being perfect? Why is it so wrong to get things wrong or make a mistake?

Try aiming to be 'good enough' rather than perfect. At the same time, check your boundaries. Just because you have had a need to be perfect, why should others live by your rules?

To make the switch from wanting to be perfect to being merely 'good enough' – that is, neither perfect nor hopeless – and to occupy that middle ground instead is hard. Change is always difficult, but just because it's hard doesn't mean you should stop trying.

Expect that it will be difficult. Expect that it will feel strange to try to be merely 'good enough' and to expect others to be 'good enough', too, rather than perfect. Learn to tolerate being in the middle, 'good enough' ground. The more you experience this, the more comfortable it will feel and the pressure to be perfect will reduce.

Congratulate yourself on every small success you make to stay in the middle ground.

Check your boundaries

If you feel that you are a control freak and/or others do, too, then chances are you are constantly stepping over a boundary where you in some way try to run or influence other people's lives.

When did this start? Did others step over *your* boundaries once? If they did, it probably wasn't very nice for you.

What beliefs underpin your stepping over other people's boundaries? Many people believe that they're right about things or like to do things a certain way, but they don't force others to change their views or behaviour. Do you step over the line because others allow it and it makes you feel good because they can't or don't stand up for themselves? Do you step over the line because it's an ingrained pattern of behaviour?

How can you pull back and stay on your side of the boundary? The key is simple. It's about respect. You probably expect others to respect you. If you're honest, do you expect respect yourself, but are less skilled at giving respect to others? What could you do about this?

Make the most of the support you have

Make the most of good friends and family. Accept their help and support, listen to their advice.

Become part of something that you sense will offer you support – whether it's a church group or a club connected with a sport you're interested in.

Adopt a positive outlook

This might sound like a cliché, but it does help if you can look on the 'bright side'.

Smile more often. Read the newspapers so you know what's going on in the world and can see your own problems in a wider context.

Stop blaming yourself for past mistakes. Start today.

Respect others' rights to be different from you

Do you respect that others have a right to be different from you, that they're entitled to hold different views and opinions and have different needs and wishes from yours? Also, crucially, that being different from you and holding different views, opinions, needs, wants, desires and wanting to do things differently, not liking the same people or not having the same mood as you at the same time does not mean that they disrespect you, and that these things do not diminish you in any way.

Being able to tolerate that people are different from you is a sign of emotional intelligence and maturity. If you find it difficult to tolerate differences like these, how can you change that?

Try to cultivate a sense of curiosity about your partner (and everyone else). Being curious about people, about what makes them tick, why they are the way they are, and developing an interest in how they are different from you, is the polar opposite of expecting or demanding that people are just like you and want to do things exactly as you would do them, or see things exactly as you see them. It's also a much more interesting way to live your life, to be curious about other people and open to their differences, instead of starting with a rigid list of expectations they have to meet.

Accept that people change their minds. Their views and their needs and wishes change, too. It's the same for others as it is for you. No one stays the same. Wouldn't life be dull if they did? Have a go at being more open to what *is*, rather than needing to stick to what you think *should* happen. Accept that other people can and do and are entitled to change their minds and that's their business.

Consider talking through and signing up to a 'bill of rights', such as the one below, with your partner, so you are both working to the same set of 'rules'. This will help to ensure that you respect each other more and stick to your boundaries.

So, what are your respective rights? I would offer the following list, but you might want to add some of your own. Notice what you feel when you read them. Do you sense that it would feel good if these rules applied to you but not to your partner? What does that tell you? What could you do about it?

Bill of 21 Rights

The following list was inspired by and adapted from *A Woman in Your Own Right* by Anne Dickson (1982).

1 I have the right to take care of myself.
2 I have the right to state my own needs and decide my own priorities.
3 I have the right to make my own decisions.
4 I have the right to have and state my own views.
5 I have the right to be respected as an individual.

6   I have the right to be treated with respect as an equal human being.

7   I have the right to express my own feelings.

8   I have the right *not* to be perfect.

9   I have the right to say 'yes' or 'no' to requests and have my decisions respected.

10   I have the right to make mistakes.

11   I have the right to change my mind.

12   I have the right to privacy.

13   I have the right to determine what I choose to do or not do with my own body.

14   I have the right to ask for what I want or need.

15   I have the right to say 'I don't understand'.

16   I have the right to get things wrong.

17   I have the right to take responsibility for my own actions.

18   I have the right to *not* have to take responsibility for other people's actions.

19   I have the right to decide and determine my own future.

20   I have the right to say 'no'.

21   I have the right to do what I need to so that I can maintain self-respect, providing this does not involve harming or abusing others.

Accept some hard and bitter truths

Some bits of life are unpleasant. Things don't always go the way we want them to. It can help if you accept some uncomfortable truths. These are, of course, my truths. They may not be yours, but see what you think.

- Your truth, your version of events, may be completely different from someone else's version, but that doesn't necessarily mean one of you is wrong. You could *both* be right because people see things differently. People notice different things. People feel different things ... and that's all right.
- You don't always get and can't always have what you think you deserve.
- You can't inoculate yourself against loss, suffering, unfairness or insecurity. It's a fact of life that bad stuff happens and sometimes we learn masses from it.
- You can't always eliminate all anxiety, risk, negative feelings or other bad stuff from your life, but you can learn to live with it positively in a different way. By accepting it, you may help to eliminate it.

- You can't control everything; but by giving up the need for control, you might end up feeling more in control!

Mindfulness meditation and how it might help you

Mindfulness meditation is not the same as relaxing or visualizing a restful scene, though you may find that helpful. In a way, it's the exact opposite of relaxation.

Mindfulness is the art of learning to be aware, moment to moment, non-judgementally and with curiosity, so you have more choices about how you react to thoughts. It can help you to 'get in the gap' between a thought and action. So, instead of having a thought and ending up in a downward spiral of negativity, you can tell yourself that it's 'just a thought', not a fact, and learn to tolerate having the thought without it leading to further negative thoughts or controlling behaviours.

Mindfulness meditation is part of a therapy being used in the UK that is also popular in the USA, called mindfulness-based cognitive therapy (MBCT), which is mentioned in the NICE guidelines as being effective in helping prevent recurrent depression. It's becoming clear that it has many other applications, too. I've found it can be very useful for clients who, for example, experience jealousy of their partners, have OCD or are controlling in a variety of ways.

It is different from cognitive behaviour therapy (CBT). CBT teaches that if you can change your thoughts, then you can change your feelings. MBCT, however, teaches that thoughts are, well, just thoughts! You don't have to distract yourself from them and you don't have to act on them either. You can just observe that they're thoughts and let them pass you by, or make a different choice about what you do with them.

Mindfulness exercises can help you to be more in touch with the present moment, rather than dwell on the past or worry about the future. The idea is that the more aware you are, the more choices you have. Negative thoughts are incredibly powerful: they can lead to anxiety, depression or anger, because we rarely stop to question our thoughts. Most of us work on the assumption that, because we have a thought, then it must be true! Then one thought leads to another ... By practising being more 'in the moment' and developing your awareness so that you actually notice your thoughts before they 'take hold', and learning to treat them simply as thoughts, rather than facts, you can prevent yourself from being dragged down into a negative thought process.

The idea is not that you try to control your thoughts – a great antidote for self-confessed control freaks in itself – but the opposite.

You learn to relax and take the attitude of 'let them come, whatever thoughts they are' because you now know that thoughts can't hurt you. So, even if you continue to have *exactly the same kinds of thoughts that you have at the moment*, thoughts that normally lead you to act in a controlling way or result in arguments with your partner, or make you feel anxious or depressed or dent your self-esteem, by practising mindfulness meditation, you may be able to deal with those thoughts in a much better way. They won't control you any more and, hopefully, you may feel less need to control others.

While it can be a very good idea to distract yourself if, for example, you find that you are feeling hurt or angry, mindfulness, by contrast, offers a different solution. By noticing that you feel angry (rather than just being angry – there's a difference) and bringing a sense of curiosity to how you feel, a sense of kindness and of being non-judgmental, you may, paradoxically, transform the anger so it more naturally dissipates. It's quite hard to explain – it's one of those things that you need to practise to see the benefits.

The best way to learn mindfulness meditation at home is to practise by listening to a CD. The book *The Mindful Way through Depression* by Mark Williams, John Teasdale, Zindel Segal and Jon Kabat-Zinn (2007) explains mindfulness brilliantly (you don't have to be suffering from depression to read it) and comes with a CD. Meanwhile, you might want to try the exercises below to get you started.

Exercise: Breath awareness – ten minutes every day

Sit quietly where you won't be interrupted for ten minutes a day and simply focus your attention on your breathing.

Pay attention to the physical sensations of breathing and be fully aware of each in-breath and each out-breath. Don't try to control the breath in any way, just be aware of it. Other thoughts may pop into your mind or you may become distracted by sounds. When that happens, just note each one in your mind non-judgementally and then bring your attention back to the sensation of the breath.

That's all you have to do. Keep bringing your attention back to the breath. Don't worry about distractions – it is just as valuable to become aware that the mind has wandered as it is to be able to stay aware and focus on the breath. That is because, if you become aware your mind has wandered, then you are exactly that – *aware*, you're not on autopilot.

So, don't beat yourself up or think you're 'doing it wrong' because you realize that your mind has wandered. Congratulate yourself for having noticed, then gently bring your attention back to the breath.

It's also extremely valuable to do this exercise for just one or three minutes at odd times during the day on top of the ten minutes. It sounds easy, but you may find it hard at first and it may seem pointless. Trust that it is not pointless and could help you.

You might want to see this exercise as a 'safe harbour' – something you can easily do at other times if you feel stressed – and trust that it will help you feel better.

Remember, you're not trying to control your thoughts but learning to actually feel comfortable with letting things be *as they already are*, whatever that happens to be, then returning to the breath. This will help you tolerate uncomfortable feelings and situations – such as when things aren't going the way you want – and make better choices in difficult situations, for example, if someone you're speaking to becomes angry.

It's important to realize that mindfulness isn't a 'technique' – it is more a helpful way of being. It sounds easy, but it does require effort to practise. Jon Kabat-Zinn says that it 'allows us to see more clearly, and therefore come to understand more deeply, areas in our lives that we were out of touch with or unwilling to look at.' It can, he says 'free us from the ruts we so often fall into. It is empowering as well because paying attention in this way opens channels to deep resources of creativity, intelligence, imagination, clarity, determination, choice and wisdom within us'. Sounds good, doesn't it!

Another benefit of mindfulness is that it can help you become better at 'letting go' (Kabat-Zinn, 2004). We often get 'stuck', unable to change our ways, views or thoughts. Mindfulness helps us become aware of where we are stuck and helps us more easily let go of familiar, but unhelpful, patterns or ways of behaving.

Exercise: Body scan practice

Bring awareness to each part of your body in turn and then 'let go' of your awareness of that part of the body before moving your attention to the next part.

This exercise is best done with the help of a CD as, at first, it can be helpful to simply listen and follow the instructions without having to remember what to do.

As with the previous exercise, it's a way of learning to be 'in the moment' rather than letting your mind race on about this, that or the other. (You'll find a useful CD in the back of the book by Mark Williams et al., 2007, mentioned above.)

Exercise: Everyday mindfulness

Find opportunities to use mindfulness in everyday activities, such as washing up, brushing your teeth, walking to the shops, mowing the lawn, having a shower and so on. Just focus wholly on what you are doing, nothing else, noticing whatever you happen to notice.

Another idea is to take a few moments out to go and look at the clouds or a flower or the stars. Notice, perhaps in a way that you never have before, what's there, what you feel, what you can see as you do this. Whether it's the patterns or textures, the feeling of the breeze on your face or whatever, the idea is that as you become generally more aware, so you begin to notice and enjoy the good bits of life more acutely than you used to.

Reading this chapter may have been hard if you have recognized yourself as being a control freak or you know that others think you are one, but I hope it will also have given you plenty of practical tips and ideas so you feel more positive about the possibility of change, if that's what you want. Also, that you'll start to have a sense of loving kindness towards yourself and a feeling of hopefulness. By becoming more aware of what you are doing and how you are feeling, taking responsibility for yourself and allowing others to take responsibility for themselves, and treating yourself and others with the same level of respect, you may begin to make different decisions and create a hopefully better future for yourself and the people around you, whom you love and who love you.

Useful addresses

These are just a few of the self-help organizations or charities in the UK that could be of assistance to you. It is worth investigating to see if there are any organizations especially for your area. A good website that enables you to search for self-help organizations nationally and locally is <www.self-help.org.uk>. See also <www.bacp.co.uk>. Bear in mind that, over time, helpline numbers change and smaller organizations cease to operate; but the following details were correct at the time of publication.

Alcohol- and drug-related help

Al-Anon
1 Great Dover Street
London SE1 4YF
Tel.: 020 7403 0888 (Helpline 10 a.m. to 10 p.m., 365 days a year)
028 9068 2368 (Northern Ireland);
01 873 2699 (Republic of Ireland);
0141 339 8884 (Helpline 10 a.m. to 10 p.m., 365 days a year: Scotland)
Website: www.al-anonuk.org.uk
Assists the friends and families of alcoholics.

Alcohol Concern
64 Leman Street
London E1 8EU
Tel.: 020 7264 0510
Website: www.alcoholconcern.org.uk

Alcohol Concern Cymru
Sophia House
28 Cathedral Road
Cardiff CF11 9LJ
Tel.: 029 2066 0248
Website: www.alcoholconcern.org.uk

Center on Addiction and the Family
50 Jay Street
Brooklyn
New York
NY 11201
USA
Tel.: 001 718 222 6641
Website: www.coaf.org
US organization offering support and information.

FRANK
Helpline: 0800 776600
Website: www.talktofrank.com
Charity specializing in advice and information via 24-hour helpline every day.

National Association for Children of Alcoholics
PO Box 64
Fishponds
Bristol BS16 2UH
Helpline: 0800 358 3456
Website: www.nacoa.org.uk

Boarding school

Boarding School Survivors
6 Chester Court
Lissenden Gardens
London NW5 1LY
Tel.: 020 7267 7098
Website: www. boardingschoolsurvivors.co.uk
For information and workshops on the psychological effects on children sent to boarding school.

Bullying

ACAS
Euston Tower
286 Euston Road
London NW1 3JJ
Tel. (helpline): 08457 474747
(8 a.m. to 8 p.m., Monday to
Friday; 9 a.m. to 1 p.m., Saturday)
Website: www.acas.org.uk
Provides advice to both employers
and employees who are involved
in an employment dispute or
who are seeking information on
employment rights.

Andrea Adams Trust
Shalimar House
24 Derek Avenue
Hove
East Sussex BN3 4PF
Tel.: 01273 389412
Website: www.andreaadamstrust.org
www.banbullyingatwork.com
Offers training and consultancy help
for those who have experienced
bullying in the workplace.

Bully OnLine
Website: www.bullyonline.org
Provides assistance for those
experiencing bullying in general,
e.g. in the workplace, at home,
in school, etc., and help and
information on issues related to
bullying.

National Bullying Helpline
15 Dorcan Business Village
Murdock Road
Swindon SN3 5HY
Tel.: 0845 2255 787 (helpline: 10
a.m. to 4 p.m., Monday to Friday;
10 a.m. to 2 p.m., Saturday)
Website: www.nationalbullyinghelp
line.co.uk

Counselling and Relationships

**British Association for
Counselling and Psychotherapy**
BACP House
15 St John's Business Park
Lutterworth
Leics LE17 4HB
Tel.: 01455 883300
Website: www.bacp.co.uk
Professional body for counsellors
and psychotherapists; holds
the United Kingdom Register of
Counsellors and Psychotherapists;
log on to find a suitable and
accredited therapist near you.

Co-dependents Anonymous
Website: www.coda-uk.org
Informal self-help groups made up
of men and women with a common
interest in working through the
problems that codependency
has caused in their lives. CODA's
programme of recovery is based
on that of Alcoholics Anonymous,
i.e. it involves attending meetings
and working through the 12-step
programme.

Couples Counselling Network
Website: www.
ukcouplescounselling.com
Portal for finding a counsellor
specializing in couple counselling.

Institute of Transactional Analysis
Broadway House
149–151 St Neots Road
Hardwick
Cambridge CB23 7QJ
Tel.: 0845 0099 101
Website: www.ita.org.uk
For those interested in the work of
Eric Berne and who would like to
find a TA therapist.

Relate
Premier House
Carolina Court
Lakeside
Doncaster DN4 5RA
Tel.: 0300 100 1234
Website: www.relate.org.uk
For people seeking relationship
counselling.

**United Kingdom Register of
Counsellors and Psychotherapists**
Tel.: 01455 883300
Website: www.ukrconline.org.uk
For further details, see **British
Association for Counselling and
Psychotherapy** above.

Depression

Depression Alliance
212 Spitfire Studios
63–71 Collier Street
London N1 9BE
Tel.: 020 8760 0544 (office)
Information pack request line: 0845
123 2320
Website: www.
depressionalliance.org
Leading UK charity for people
affected by depression.

Depression Alliance Scotland
1 Alva Street
Edinburgh EH2 4PH
Tel.: 0131 467 3050 (see above for
info pack request line)
Website: www.dascot.org

Journeys (formerly **Depression
Alliance Cymru**)
120–122 Broadway
Roath
Cardiff CF24 1NJ
Tel.: 029 2069 2891
Website: www.journeysonline.org.uk

Mental health

**Centre for Anxiety Disorders and
Trauma**
Website: http://psychology.iop.kcl.
ac.uk/cadat/
Useful website for information
about post-traumatic stress disorder
(PTSD) and other topics.

Combat Stress
Chief Executive
Tyrwhitt House
Oaklawn Road
Leatherhead
Surrey KT22 0BX
Tel.: 01372 841600
Website: www.combatstress.org.uk
Assists ex-servicemen and women
suffering from stress-related mental
illness.

Living Life to the Full
Website:
www.livinglifetothefull.com
Online cognitive behaviour
therapy (CBT) course devised by
Dr Chris Williams, senior lecturer
in psychiatry at the University of
Glasgow. This programme is free
and is widely recommended by GPs
and counsellors.

MIND (National Association for
Mental Health)
15–19 Broadway
Stratford
London E15 4BQ
Tel.: 020 8519 2122
Mind*info*Line: 0845 766 0163
Website: www.mind.org.uk
Provides support for people in
mental distress and their families
through advice, campaigns and
local services. There are more than
200 local groups in England and
Wales.

Mind Cymru (Wales)
Third Floor, Quebec House
Castlebridge
5–19 Cowbridge Road East
Cardiff CF11 9AB
Tel.: 029 2039 5123
Website: www.mind.org.uk

Mindfulness-Based Cognitive Therapy (MBCT)
Wellcome Building
University of Oxford Department of Psychiatry
Warneford Hospital
Oxford OX3 7JX
Website: www.mbct.co.uk (UK)
www.mbct.com (worldwide)
The UK website is attached to the University of Oxford and provides information, resources, CDs, etc. about this particular branch of psychotherapy first developed in the USA. The worldwide website offers similar resources.

National Personality Disorder Programme
Website: www.personalitydisorder.org.uk
Provides information and resources about personality disorders.

No Panic
93 Brands Farm Way
Telford
Shropshire TF3 2JQ
Tel.: 01952 590005
Helpline: 0808 808 0545
Website: www.nopanic.org.uk
Offers advice on phobias, panic attacks and obsessive–compulsive disorder (OCD).

OCD-UK
PO Box 8955
Nottingham NG10 9AU
Tel.: 0845 120 3778 (for general enquiries: not a helpline. Voice messages will be answered.)
Website: www.ocduk.org
OCD-UK is a new national charity, which has been founded for people who are affected by obsessive–compulsive disorder (OCD).

Paranoid Thoughts
Website: http://www.iop.kcl.ac.uk/apps/paranoidthoughts/default.aspx
A resource to assist those distressed by thoughts of this kind.

PsychCentral
Website: http://psychcentral.com
This US website contains online articles and resources about mental health, relationships etc.

Rethink
89 Albert Embankment
London SE1 7TP
Tel.: 0845 456 0455 (general)
National advice service: 020 7840 3188 (10 a.m. to 1 p.m., Monday to Friday)
Website: www.rethink.org
Provides an information service for people with mental health problems.

Royal College of Psychiatrists
17 Belgrave Square
London SW1X 8PG
Tel.: 020 7235 2351
Website: www.rcpsych.ac.uk
The main professional organization of psychiatrists in the UK, the College provides, among a wide range of resources, online self-help leaflets on common mental health problems.

Samaritans
Chris
PO Box 9090
Stirling FK8 2SA
Tel.: 08457 90 90 90
Website: www.samaritans.org
Provides confidential, emotional
support for all those in distress, 24
hours a day. Telephone directories
list local branches.

SANE
First Floor, Cityside House
40 Adler Street
London E1 1EE
Tel.: 020 7375 1002 (general
enquiries)
SANEline: 0845 767 8000 (national
helpline for people and/or their
carers affected by mental health
problems, open 6 p.m. to 11 p.m.
daily)
Website: www.sane.org.uk
This charity offers emotional
support and information on all
aspects of mental health.

Psychological and violent abuse

Everyman Project
1A Waterlow Road
London N19 5NJ
Tel.: 020 7263 8884 (advice line)
Website: www.
everymanproject.co.uk
Offers a range of support services
for men who want to stop behaving
violently or abusively, and for their
partners.

Men's Advice Line
Tel.: 0808 801 0327 (10 a.m. to 1
p.m./2 p.m. to 5 p.m., Monday to
Friday)
Website: www.
mensadviceline.org.uk
Managed by **Respect** (see below),
this line provides advice and
support for men in abusive
relationships.

Refuge
2–8 Maltravers Street
London WC2R 3EE
Tel.: 020 7395 7700 (office)
Helpline: see **Women's Aid** (on the
facing page)
Website: www.refuge.org.uk
This charity provides emergency
accommodation for women and
children fleeing domestic violence,
and emotional and practical
support, including a list of pet-
fostering services when partners
threaten the welfare of a pet.

Respect
First Floor, 1 Downstream Building
1 London Bridge
London SE1 9BG
Tel.: 020 7022 1801 (office)
Phoneline: 0845 122 8609 (10 a.m.
to 1 p.m. and 2 to 5 p.m., Monday
to Friday)
Website: www.respect.uk.net or
www.respectphoneline.org.uk
This UK membership association
runs programmes for those who
perpetrate domestic violence
and support services for those
experiencing violence. It also
manages the **Men's Advice Line.**

Shelter
88 Old Street
London EC1V 9HU
Free housing advice helpline: 0808
800 444
Website: www.shelter.org.uk/
National charity for housing and
homelessness.

Women's Aid
Women's Aid Federation of
England Head Office
PO Box 391
Bristol BS99 7WS
Freephone National Domestic
Violence Helpline: 0808 2000 247
(24 hours a day)
Website: www.womensaid.org.uk
National charity working to end
domestic violence against women
and children.

Women's Aid (Scottish)
Second Floor, 132 Rose Street
Edinburgh EH2 3JD
Domestic Abuse Helpline: 0800 027
1234 (24 hours a day)
Website: www.
scottishwomensaid.org.uk

Women's Aid (Welsh)
38–48 Crwys Road
Cardiff CF24 4NN
Domestic Abuse Helpline: 0808 80
10 800 (24 hours a day)
Website: www.welshwomensaid.org

References and further reading

Aguilar, R. J., and Nightingale, N. N. (1994) 'The impact of specific battering experiences on the self-esteem of abused women', *Journal of Family Violence*, 9, 33–45

American Psychiatric Association (2000) *Diagnostic and Statistical Manual of Mental Disorders* (4th edn), Washington, DC, American Psychiatric Association

Arias, I., and Pape, Karen T. (1999) 'Psychological abuse: implications for adjustment and commitment to leave violent partners' in D. O'Leary and R. D. Maiuro (2001) *Psychological Abuse in Violent Domestic Relations*, New York, Springer

Baldry, A. C. (2003) 'Sticks and stones hurt my bones but his glance and words hurt more: the impact of psychological abuse and physical violence by current and former partners on battered women in Italy', *International Journal of forensic Mental Health*, 2 (1), pp. 47–57

Bursten, B. (1973) 'Some narcissistic personality types', *International Journal of Psychoanalysis*, 53, pp. 287–300

Cobb, J. P. and Marks I. M. (1979) 'Morbid jealousy featuring an obsessive–compulsive neurosis: treatment by behavioural psychotherapy', *The British Journal of Psychiatry*, 134, pp. 301–5

Docherty, J. P., and Ellis, J. (1976) 'A new concept and finding in morbid jealousy', *American Journal of Psychiatry*, 133, pp. 679–83

Dutton, D. G., and Painter, S. (1993) 'Emotional attachments in abusive relationships: a test of traumatic bonding theory', *Violence and Victims*, 8, pp. 105–20

Enoch, M. D., and Trethowan, W. J. (1979) *Uncommon Psychiatric Syndromes* (2nd edn), Bristol, John Wright, cited in M. Kingham and H. Gordon (2004) 'Aspects of morbid jealousy', *Advances in Psychiatric Treatment*, 10, pp. 207–15

Fennig, S., Fochtmann, L. J., Bromet, E. J. (2005) 'Delusional and shared psychotic disorder' in B. J. Sadock and V. A. Sadock (eds), *Kaplan & Sadock's Comprehensive Textbook of Psychiatry* (8th edn), Philadelphia, PA, Lippincott Williams & Wilkins, pp. 1525–33

Follingstad, D. R., Rutledge, L. L., Berg, B. J., Hause, E. S., and Polek, D. S. (1990) 'The role of emotional abuse in physically abusive relationships', *Journal of Family Violence*, 5, pp. 107–20

Freeman, D. (2006) 'Delusions in the non-clinical population', *Current Psychiatry Reports*, 8, pp. 191–204

Graham, D. L. R., with Rawlings, E. I., and Rigsby, R. (1994) *Loving to Survive: Sexual terror, men's violence and women's lives*, New York, New York University Press

Home Office (2009) 'Together we can end violence against women and girls', a consultation paper, Home Office (also available online at <www. homeoffice.gov.uk/documents/cons-2009-vaw/>)

Jarrett, C. (2006) 'Understanding personality disorder', *The Psychologist*, 19 (7), pp. 402–4

Kahler, T. (1975) 'Scripts: process and content', *Transactional Analysis*, 5 (3), pp. 277–79

Kingham, M., and Gordon, H. (2004) 'Aspects of morbid jealousy', *Advances in Psychiatric Treatment*, 10, pp. 207–15

Marazziti, D., Di Nasso, E., Masala, I., Baroni, S., Abelli, M., Mengali, F., Mungai, F., and Rucci, P. (2003) 'Normal and obsessional jealousy: a study of a population of young adults', *European Psychiatry*, 18 (3), pp. 106–11

Marshall, L. L. (1996) 'Psychological abuse of women: six distinct clusters', *Journal of Family Violence*, 11, pp. 379–409

Marshall, Linda L. (2001) 'Effects of men's subtle and overt psychological abuse on low-income women' in D. O'Leary and R. D. Maiuro (2001) *Psychological Abuse in Violent Domestic Relations*, New York, Springer

Michael, A., Mirza, S., Mirza, K. A. H., Babu, V. S. and Vithayathil, E. (1995) 'Morbid jealousy in alcoholism', *British Journal of Psychiatry*, 167, pp. 668–72, cited in M. Kingham and H. Gordon (2004) 'Aspects of morbid jealousy', *Advances in Psychiatric Treatment*, 10, pp. 207–15

'National Workplace Bullying Survey 2005', Digital Opinion/Personnel Today and the Andrea Adams Trust, available online at <www.digita-lopinion.co.uk/bullying-natsurvey-results.html>

O'Leary, D .K. (2001) 'Psychological abuse: a variable deserving critical attention in domestic violence' in D. O'Leary and R. D. Maiuro, *Psychological Abuse in Violent Domestic Relations*, New York, Springer

O'Leary, D., and Maiuro, R. D. (2001) *Psychological Abuse in Violent Domestic Relations*, New York, Springer

Parker, G. (1997) 'Morbid jealousy as a variant of obsessive–compulsive disorder', *Australian and New Zealand Journal of Psychiatry*, 31 (1), pp. 133–8

Sims, A. (1995) *Symptoms in the Mind* (2nd edn), London, W. B. Saunders, cited in M. Kingham and H. Gordon (2004) 'Aspects of morbid jealousy', *Advances in Psychiatric Treatment*, 10, pp. 207–15

Veale, D. (2002) 'Over-valued ideas: a conceptual analysis', *Behaviour Research and Therapy*, 40 (4), pp. 383–400

White, G. L., and Mullen, P. E. (1989) *Jealousy: Theory, research and clinical strategies*, New York, Guilford Press

Of interest to therapists

Beck, Aaron T., Freeman, Arthur, Davis, Denise D. and associates (2007) *Cognitive Therapy of Personality Disorders*, New York, Guilford Press

Beck, Judith S. (2005) *Cognitive Therapy for Challenging Problems*, New York, Guilford Press

O'Leary, K. Daniel, and Maiuro, Roland D. (eds) (2004) *Psychological Abuse in Violent Domestic Relations*, New York, Springer

Parker Hall, Sue (2008) *Anger Rage and Relationship: An empathic approach to anger management*, Abingdon, Routledge

Segal, Zindel, Williams, Mark, and Teasdale, John (2002) *Mindfulness-based Cognitive Therapy for Depression: A new approach to preventing relapse*, New York, Guilford Press

Vaknin, Sam (1999) *Malignant Self Love: Narcissism revisited*, Czech Republic, Narcissus Publications

van Deurzen, Emmy, and Arnold-Baker, Claire (eds) (2005) *Existential Perspectives on Human Issues: A handbook for therapeutic practice*, Basingstoke, Palgrave Macmillan

Mindfulness

Brantley, Jeffrey (2007) *Calming Your Anxious Mind: How mindfulness and compassion can free you from anxiety, fear and panic* (2nd rev. edn), Oakland, CA, New Harbinger Publications

Kabat-Zinn, Jon (2004) *Wherever You Go, There You Are*, London, Piatkus

Williams, Mark, Teasdale, John, Segal, Zindel and Kabat-Zinn, Jon (2007) *The Mindful Way through Depression*, New York, Guilford Press (comes with a CD to help you practise)

Personality disorders

Alwin, N., Blackburn, R., Davidson, K., Hilton, M., Logan C. D., and Shine, J. (2006) *Understanding Personality Disorder: A report by the British Psychological Society*, Leicester, British Psychological Society (also available online at <www.bps.org.uk>, click Media Centre, then Press Releases, 2006, page 5)

Masterson, James F. (1993) *The Search For the Real Self*, New York, Free Press

Phillipson, Steven (no date) 'The RIGHT stuff: obsessive compulsive personality disorder: a defect of philosophy, not anxiety', available online at <www.ocdonline.com>, click on Articles by Dr Steven Phillipson

Self-help

Baker, Barbara (2003) *When Someone You Love has Depression*, London, Sheldon Press

Beattie, Melody (2009) *The New Codependency: Help and guidance for today's generation*, London, Simon & Schuster

Beck, Aaron T. (1988) *Love is Never Enough: How couples can overcome misunderstandings, resolve conflicts and solve relationship problems through cognitive therapy*, London, HarperCollins

Berne, Eric (2004) *Games People Play: The psychology of human relationships*, London, Penguin

Clark, David, and Purdon, Christine (2009) *Overcoming Obsessive Thoughts:*

How to gain control of your OCD, Oakland, CA, New Harbinger Publications

Davies, William (2000) *Overcoming Anger and Irritability: A self-help guide using cognitive behavioural techniques*, London, Robinson

Dickson, Anne (1982) *A Woman In Your Own Right: Assertiveness and you*, London, Quartet

Dryden, Windy (2005) *Overcoming Jealousy*, London, Sheldon Press

Dryden, Windy, and Constantinou, Daniel (2004) *Assertiveness Step by Step*, London, Sheldon Press

Elliot-Wright, Susan (2008) *Overcoming Insomnia: How to sleep like a dream*, London, Sheldon Press

Fennell, Melanie (2009) *Overcoming Low Self-esteem: A self-help guide using cognitive behavioral techniques*, London, Robinson

Field, Tim (1996) *Bully in Sight: How to predict, resist, challenge and combat workplace bullying*, Success Unlimited

Freeman, Daniel, Freeman, Jason and Garety, Philippa (2008) *Overcoming Paranoid and Suspicious Thoughts*, New York, Basic Books

Hartley, Mary (2002) *Managing Anger at Work*, London, Sheldon Press

Horley, Sandra (2002) *Power and Control: Why charming men can make dangerous lovers*, London, Vermilion

Kennerley, Helen (2000) *Overcoming Childhood Trauma: A self-help guide using cognitive behavioral techniques*, London, Robinson

Tallis, Dr Frank (1992) *Understanding Obsessions and Compulsions*, London, Sheldon Press

Index